BIOMEDICAL DEVICES AND THEIR APPLICATIONS

ADAPTIVE FILTERING TECHNIQUES FOR REMOTE HEALTH CARE MONITORING SYSTEMS

BIOMEDICAL DEVICES AND THEIR APPLICATIONS

Additional books and e-books in this series can be found on Nova's website under the Series tab.

Biomedical Devices and their Applications

Adaptive Filtering Techniques for Remote Health Care Monitoring Systems

Zia Ur Rahman, PhD

nova
Medicine & Health
New York

Additional color graphics may be available in the e-book version of this book.

Library of Congress Cataloging-in-Publication Data

ISBN: 978-1-53614-749-0
Library of Congress Control Number: 2018965003

Published by Nova Science Publishers, Inc. † New York

CONTENTS

LIST OF FIGURES

List of Tables

PREFACE

Adaptive Filtering Techniques for Remote Health Care Monitoring Systems aims to present a full picture of the state-of-the art research and development of adaptive filtering techniques in telecardiology applications. This book covers the broad investigations and analysis of adaptive filters in remote health care monitoring to remove various artifacts as well as channel noise encountered in transmission. The ability to extract high resolution, valid ECG signals from contaminated recordings is an important subject for research.

In remote cardiac diagnosis, telecardiology has becomes an important tool enabling the transmission of electrocardiogram (ECG) signals between widely separated locations. Received signals can be recorded and processed to allow diagnosis so that the specialist can advise the patient. However, during ECG acquisition several artifacts strongly degrade the signal quality. The dominant artifacts encounter with ECG signal are Power Line Interference (PLI), Baseline Wander (BW), Muscle Artifacts (MA), Electrode Motion Artifacts (EM) and channel noise generated during transmission. All of these masks the tiny features of ECG signal that specialists depend upon for clinical monitoring, interpretation and diagnosis. The ability to extract high resolution, valid ECG signals from contaminated recordings is an important subject for research. In practice, contaminated cardiac signals are non-stationary and fixed coefficient filters will not work well. To track random variations in noisy signals, the filter has to be adaptive, able to change its coefficients according to the statistical nature of the noise. This work investigates the development of Adaptive Noise Cancellers (ANCs) to remove artifacts from ECG signals.

Complexity reduction of the noise cancellation system, particularly, in applications such as biotelemetry system has been remained a topic of intense research. This is because increasing the number of data samples transmitted causes them to overlap when received. This drawback can be overcome by reducing the computational complexity of the adaptive filter. To cope with both the complexity and the convergence issues without any restrictive trade-off, we propose various simpler ANCs for ECG denoising. To achieve this, we consider three categories of adaptive algorithms: weight updates variants of the basic Least Mean Square (LMS) adaptive algorithm; normalized adaptive algorithms; and block adaptive algorithms.

In the first phase, we developed ANCs using weight update variants of the LMS algorithm. To reduce the computational complexity, we extended these algorithms by combining them with sign algorithms. These algorithms require less computational complexity than LMS algorithm, so are good candidates for practical implementation.

Next, we considered normalized version of the LMS algorithm to improve the convergence speed. By combining data, error normalization with sign algorithms, we designed ANCs with fast convergence, low computational complexity and large signal to noise ratio, all parameters greatly required in biotelemetry system.

Our third category, block adaptive algorithms, recognizes the requirement for extremely long adaptive filters to cope with the large number of samples in the signals transmitted in real time applications. In cases like these, block processing can significantly reduce the computational complexity of adaptive filters, as filtering is accomplished through block by block processing of data samples. Using this strategy, we developed several ANCs based on block processing in time and frequency domains.

Using MATLAB and the techniques described above, we developed 42 ANCs to remove artifacts from ECG signals. To study the performance of the filter structures, we carried out simulation studies at the MIT-BIH database under different noise conditions. The eight best performers ANCs are considered for real time implementation of an embedded processor, TI TMS320C6713 DSP, rewritten from MATLAB to C language. For standardization, the experimental results were compared with those obtained from a conventional LMS based noise canceller. The experimental results fit well with simulation results and are presented in this work.

It is certainly not the author's ambition to cover everything concerning adaptive filtering principles and applications. Rather, this book features the various classifications of adaptive algorithms in the contest of cardiac signal enhancement for a typical remote health care monitoring system. Another important aspect addressed in this book is computational complexity. Complexity reduction of the noise cancellation system, particularly, in applications such as biotelemetry system has been remained a topic of intense research. This is because increasing the number of data samples transmitted causes them to overlap when received. This drawback can be overcome by reducing the computational complexity of the adaptive filter. All the algorithms are analyzed in ECG enhancement process and several algorithms are also tested on an embedded processor, to validate the performance of the techniques suitable for real time applications.

The intended audience of this book will mainly consist of researchers, research students and practitioners in adaptive filtering and applications. This book is also of interest to researchers and industrial practitioners in areas such as algorithm developers, biomedical engineers, biomedical instrumentation, machine learning, and artificial intelligence. This book will present research outcomes on theoretical and technical issues related to real time application.

ABBREVIATIONS

ADC	Analog to digital conversion
ANC	Adaptive Noise Canceller
APA	Affine Projection Algorithm
ASC	Addition with Sign Check
BB	Block Based
BBENLMS	Block Based ENLMS
BBENSLMS	Block Based ENSLMS
BBENSRLMS	Block Based ENSRLMS
BBENSSLMS	Block Based ENSSLMS
BBNLMS	Block Based NLMS
BBNSLMS	Block Based NSLMS
BBNSRLMS	Block Based NSRLMS
BBNSSLMS	Block Based NSSLMS
BENLMS	Block Error normalized LMS
BLMS	Block LMS
BNLMS	Block normalized LMS
BW	Baseline Wander
CCS	Code Composer Studio
CPR	Cardiopulmonary Resuscitation
CVD	Cardiovascular disease
DA	Distributed Arithmetic

DAC	Digital to analog conversion
DBs	Decibels
DSP	Digital Signal Processor
DSK	DSP Starter Kit
DZLMS	Dead-Zone LMS
ECG	Electrocardiogram
EM	Electrode Motion artifacts
EMG	Electromyograph
EMI	Electromagnetic Interference
EMSE	Excess Mean Square Error
ENLMS	Error Non Linear LMS algorithm
ENSLMS	Error Nonlinear Sign LMS
ENSRLMS	Error Nonlinear Signed Regressor LMS
ENSSLMS	Error Nonlinear Sign-Sign LMS
EP	Evoked Potentials
EWC	Error Whitening Criterion
FBLMS	Fast block LMS
FBENLMS	Fast BENLMS
FBNLMS	Fast BNLMS
FFT	Fast Fourier transform
FLMS	Fast LMS
FPGA	Field Programmable Gate Arrays
HR	Heart Rate
Hz.	Hertz
ICG	Impedance Cardiography
IDE	Integrated Development Environment
LA	Left Atrium
LMS	Least Mean Square
LLMS	Leaky LMS
LMF	Least Mean Fourth
LV	Left Ventricle
M_{ad}	Misadjustment
MA	Muscle Artifacts
MAC	Multiply and Accumulate

MLMS	Median LMS
MSE	Mean Square Error
NLMS	Normalized LMS
NSAF	Normalized Sub-band Adaptive Filter
NSLMS	Normalized Sign LMS
NSRDB	Normal Sinus Rhythm Database
NSRLMS	Normalized Signed Regressor LMS
NSSLMS	Normalized Sign–Sign LMS
NSTDB	Noise Stress Test Database
PDAs	Personal Digital Assistants
PLI	Power Line Interference
PNLMS	Proportionate NLMS
RA	Right Atrium
REW	Recursive Error Whitening
RLS	Recursive Least Squares
RV	Right Ventricle
SA	Sign Algorithm
SDZLMS	Signed DZLMS
SLLMS	Sign Leaky LMS
SNR	Signal to Noise Ratio
SNRI	Signal to Noise Ratio Improvement
SRA	Signed Regressor Algorithm
SRLLMS	Sign Regressor Leaky LMS
SRDZLMS	Sign Regressor DZLMS
SSA	Sign - Sign Algorithm
SSDZLMS	Sign Sign DZLMS
SSLLMS	Sign Sign Leaky LMS
TI	Texas Instruments
VSSNLMS	Variable Step Size NLMS
VLIW	Very-long-instruction-word
W-ECG	Wearable ECG Recorders

SYMBOLS

n_1	Noise in the ECG signal
n_2	Reference Noise
X (n)	Input data sample of n-the index
L	Filter length
w(n)	Tap weight vector at n-th index
$y(n)$	Filter output at n-th index
$e(n)$	Output Error at n-th index
$d(n)$	Desired response at n-th index
ξ	Mean square error
μ	Step Size parameter
γ	Leakage parameter in Leaky LMS algorithm
Sign{.}	Signum function
E[.]	Expected value of the variable in the argument
$\mu(n)$	Normalized Step size in NLMS algorithm
ε	A small constant in the denominator of $\mu(n)$
$\beta(n)$	Normalized Step size in ENLMS algorithm
P	Block length in BLMS algorithm
E (j)	Transform of the error signal vector
Z	Set of all integers
Z^{-1}	Unit delay operator

Chapter 1

INTRODUCTION

1.1. INTRODUCTION

Cardiovascular disease (CVD) refers to a large number of medical conditions relating to the heart functionality. These medical conditions relate to the abnormal health conditions that directly affecting the heart and all its components. The World health organization [143, 146] reports that, every year, millions of people in this industrialized world suffer CVDs because they are not treated promptly. Among the CVDs, heart failure is caused by the inability of the heart to pump enough blood to meet the body's need and sudden heart attacks occur when normal blood circulation ceases because the heart fails contract effectively. When the patient is far from specialist help, biotelemetry is an effective tool for the diagnosis of cardiac abnormalities [163, 164]. The cardiac signal, also called the electrocardiogram (ECG) signal is extracted by a wearable acquisition device and sent through a biotelemetry system to the hospital. There a doctor analyze the signal and decides on what action to be taken, the decision sent to the patient site for immediate action [181, 182].

In a clinical environment during acquisition the ECG signal encounters with various types of artifacts. The commonly occurred artifacts are power line interference (PLI), baseline wander (BW), muscle artifacts (MA) and electrode motion artifact (EM). These artifacts strongly affect the signal quality, which is very important for clinical monitoring, diagnosis and making their efficient cancellation imperative. Therefore the extraction of high resolution ECG signals from recordings contaminated with background noise is an important issue for investigating. The goal of ECG signal enhancement by filtering is to separate the valid signal components from the undesired artifacts, so as to present an ECG that facilitates easy and accurate interpretation.

Filtering is used to process a signal either to enhance the signal to noise ratio (SNR) or to eliminate noise of a certain type. When no a priori information is available or when the signal or noise or both are non-stationary, fixed coefficient filters cannot work effectively. In the same circumstances, however, adaptive filters have the innate ability to adjust their own parameters based on the incoming signal [12-30]. In a biotelemetry system, the computational complexity of the adaptive filter should be minimized, so that incoming data samples do not need to wait at the input port of the filter and overlapping of the data samples can be avoided.

Whit this in mind, the objective of this research is to obtain a better insight into the problem and to improve the adaptive signal processing aspects of ECG biotelemetry by developing new adaptive noise cancellers for filtering contaminated ECG signals. To achieve this, we chose three categories of adaptive signal processing algorithms as follows,

1. Weight update variants of LMS algorithm
2. Normalized adaptive algorithms
3. Block adaptive algorithms

Using these algorithms new noise cancellers for ECG enhancement are developed and presented in Chapters 3, 4 and 5 respectively.

This chapter explains the motivation behind the research, the background theory of biotelemetry, the basics of electrocardiogram signals, artifacts due to physiological and non-physiological reasons, a definition of the problem, a review of the literature on ECG enhancement and an overview of the work.

1.2. MOTIVATION

The world health organization (WHO) estimates that 17.5 million people died from cardiovascular disease (CVD) in 2005, representing 30% of all deaths worldwide [143]. If that trend continues, by 2015 more than 20 million people will die from CVD ever year [144]. In 2000, 56% of CVD deaths occurred before the age of 75. However, CVD is becoming more common in younger people, with most of the people affected now aged between 34 and 65 years [127, 145]. In addition to the fatal cases, at least 20 million people experience nonfatal heart attacks and strokes every year; many requiring continuing costly medical care [146].

CVDs can be diagnosed from the result of several different tests available for healthcare providers to look at the cardiovascular system. Dr. Robert O'Rourke et al. [184] lists the more commonly performed tests as, blood tests, ECG, chest x-ray, stress test, echocardiogram, nuclear scan, ultrasound, computed tomography (CT) scan, angiography and biopsy. Among these tests, blood tests and ECG are the primary test required. Several different blood tests may be ordered as part of evaluating someone for a cardiovascular disease. A few of these tests include: fasting glucose test, fasting lipid panel to check *cholesterol* and *triglyceride* levels, C-reactive protein (CRP) test (CRP is a blood protein that shows the presence of inflammation). One of the basic non-invasive tests are the ECG, used to assess the heart rate and rhythm. The ECG is a graphical representation of the heart's electrical activity, showing problems like abnormal heartbeats, heart damage and heart valve blockage etc. It plays a key role in cardiac patient monitoring and diagnosis. The key to treat these diseases is timely detection.

The healthcare professional chooses tests according to the patient's risk factors, history of heart problems and current symptoms. Dr. Steven Hollenberg [183] list typical symptoms indicating the need for ECG analysis required: abnormal heart beat, low heart beat shortness of breath, chest pain, rapid breathing, dizziness, loss of consciousness, weak peripheral pulse, with cold and sweating extremities and visible pallor, accompanied by hypotension, muffled heart sound. ECG analysis enables the cardiologist to identify the type of disease, for example: congestive heart failure, coronary artery disease, acute myocardial infarction, hypertension, cardiac arrhythmia and cardiomegaly [185, 186]. The ECG report provides the information on which further treatment can be decided. Advances in micro and nanotechnology have enabled the development of portable and easily operated less complicated machines. With these machines patients at remote point can easily record the ECG but diagnosis has to be done by a doctor only, who is at a far location. In practical situations such as when the patient is in the battlefield or in a remote rural location where sophisticated diagnosis is not available, if continuous monitoring of the patient is required, we make use of wireless technology.

One such technology where wireless communications utilized in health care applications is known as Biotelemetry. Biotelemetry is defined as transmitting biological or physiological data from a remote location to a location that has the capability to interpret the data and affect decision making. This includes the capability for monitoring human and animals with minimum restraint and for providing a reproduction of the transmitted data. When direct observation is impossible biotelemetry can be used to obtain the required data. In 1980 Cromwell [147] classified biotelemetry techniques two categories:

1. Bioelectrical variables, such as ECG, EMG and EEG.
2. Physiological variables that require transducers, such as blood pressure, gastrointestinal pressure, blood flow and temperature.

In 2002 N. F. Guler et al. [148] described that biomedical telemetry began as a laboratory curiosity, but that evolved in to a useful, reliable tool for data gathering. In 1903, Einthoven [147] transmitted electrocardiograms from a hospital to his laboratory by connecting immersion electrodes to a remote galvanometer directly through the telephone system, with the lines acting as conductors for the current produced by bio-potentials; modern telemetry has made a huge step forwards by eliminating wires. In 1921, Winters transmitted heart sounds over a marine radio link. External transmitters of various signals evolved as electronic technology advanced and miniaturization became possible. Later, several groups inserted small coils and electrodes into the skulls of animals. D.C. Jeutter [149] used induced alternating currents as a primitive form of telestimulation. The transmission of signals from a subject was a technique that evolved slowly until transistors were invented in the 1950, enabling signals to be transmitted from the body. The endoradiosonde, developed by Mackay and Jacobson, was one of the earliest biotelemetry units. Since the invention of integrated circuit technology in 1958, contributions of microelectronics to biomedicine and health care have been enormous. Many advanced diagnostic, therapeutic and rehabilitative devices and systems would not have been possible without these contributions. Markevitch [150] showed that signals could be transmitted through the tissues of the body from quite small coils placed within the body. Improvements in miniature and micro power are two concepts of modern biotelemetry design and construction have closely paralleled the evolution of semiconductor and micro circuit technologies. Reliable, stable integrated sensors and biotelemetry on micro circuit designs are available [151, 153].

Biotelemetry is an important method for monitoring physiological variables by providing a wireless link between the patient and the data collection equipment. Biomedical data has been telemetered through every medium between two sites, including air, space, water and biologic tissue, by using a variety of modulated energy forms like electromagnetic waves, light and ultrasound. Among these the electromagnetic waves are capable of crossing huge distances, are used in several subfields, including telemetry for medical purposes and human, animal research. Medical telemetry is of particular note because it can be used to track the vital signs of ambulatory patients remotely. In medical telemetry the potential acquired from the patient has a very low amplitude, with proper amplification and modulation it can be transmitted over a large distance. The biotelemetry system, introduced as early as the late 1950s, employs sensors, amplifiers, transmitter, a radio antenna and a receiver [148], routinely measuring parameters body temperature, heart rate, blood pressure and muscle movement.

1.2.1. Wireless Ambulatory Electrocardiogram System

One of the applications in biotelemetry is a wireless ambulatory ECG system. In which ECG signal is used as bioelectrical signal, this ECG signal is used to know the cardiac condition of an ambulatory patient. By using such wireless ambulatory system ECGs can be interpreted and treatment begun before the patient arrives at the hospital [147]. In 2004 D. Jabaudon et al. [154], and P. Chazal et al. [155] developed a microprocessor-based ECG recorders for online signal processing. A typical wireless ambulatory ECG system is shown in the Figure 1.1.

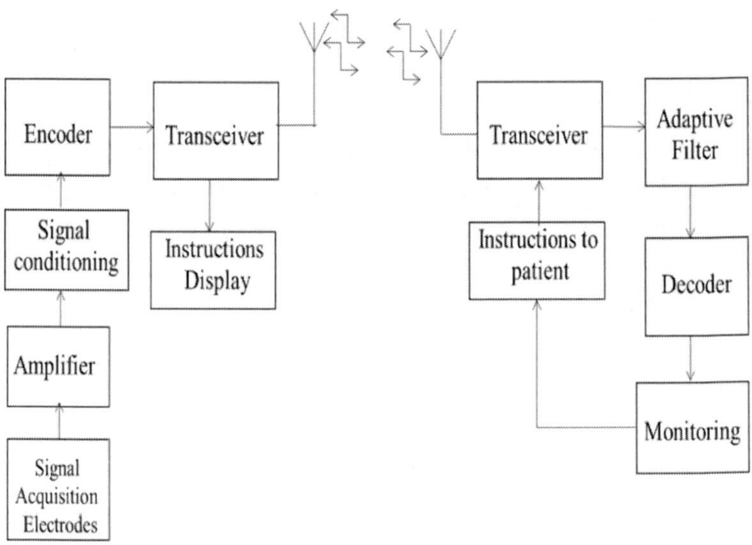

Figure 1.1. A typical wireless ambulatory ECG system.

In practice, once the ambulance arrives at the site and the patient taken on board, the ECG monitor is connected to the patient. The ECG signal is stored in the ambulance subsystem, encoded, modulated with a high frequency carrier signal and transmitted to the emergency coordination center using a GSM modem with a dedicated antenna [156]. This ECG system is facilitated with encoder and decoder at the transmitting side, receiving side. The adaptive filter used in receiving chain eliminates various artifacts and channel noise. At the emergency coordination center the clean ECG signal could be displayed for data analysis, diagnosis and sending instructions to the ambulance personnel. The paramedical people in the ambulance will thus be able to take necessary action and follow up the patients accordingly [157].

1.3. ELECTROCARDIOGRAM SIGNAL BASICS

The heart is a four chambered pump with two atria to collect blood and two ventricles to pump it out. The resting and filling phase of a cardiac chamber is called diastole, while systole is the contracting and pumping phase. The right atrium (RA) collects impure blood from the superior and inferior vena cavae. During atrial contraction, blood is passed from the RA to the right ventricle (RV) through the tricuspid valve. During ventricular systole, the impure blood in the RV is pumped out through the pulmonary valve to the lungs for purification. The left atrium (LA) receives purified blood from the lungs, which is passed on during atria contraction to the left ventricle (LV) through the mitral valve. The LV contraction is stronger as it has to pump out the oxygenated blood into the vascular system which branches throughout the body. The heart rate (HR) or cardiac rhythm is controlled by specialized pacemaker cells that form the sino-atrial (SA) node at the junction of the superior vena cava and the RA. The SA node is the basic, natural cardiac pacemaker that triggers its own train of action potentials. The action potential of the SA node propagates through the rest of the heart, causing a particular pattern of excitation and contraction, which leads to cardiac cycle [101].

An electrocardiogram (ECG) is a plot of surface bio-potential caused by the electrical activity of the cardiac muscles. It has been widely used over many years for basic cardiac monitoring in a clinical set-up. A human heart under normal conditions beats 72 times per minute, during each beat the cardiac muscles go through specifically ordered electrical activities which are distinctly identifiable from the patterns in the ECG signal. The signal is therefore very valuable for cardiac monitoring, especially as its measurement is simple, non-invasive and cost-effective. It is the primary tool for cardiac monitoring. With advances in technology, adding features like digital storage and wireless transmission of the recorded signals the ECG recording equipment is available in a smaller form. Due to this improvement, it is now practically possible to develop wearable ECG equipment for cardiac monitoring from a remote location.

Many types of cardiac disorders can be detected from the patterns in the ECG signal, especially those due to impaired electric conduction through damaged cardiac muscles. A qualified professional can identify some of the abnormal patterns visually and relate them to damages in a specific region of the heart. It is thus required to analyze signals from different leads of the ECG for determining the location of the damaged region. Here the lead refers to the signal acquired from a specific pair of ECG electrodes placed at predefined locations on the body. Thus, every ECG lead looks at the specific area of the heart and, in order to cover different areas of the heart, different ECG leads are required. The ECG equipment commonly uses the standard 12-lead configuration. The ECG signal is acquired from a pair of specific locations on the body and Ag/AgCl electrodes are used for making electrical contact with the skin surface [147]. A typical cardiac cycle (ECG beat) in the ECG signal has the following distinct characteristic segments called P wave, QRS complex and T wave occurring in a sequence are shown in Figure 1.2, which are important for in ECG analysis.

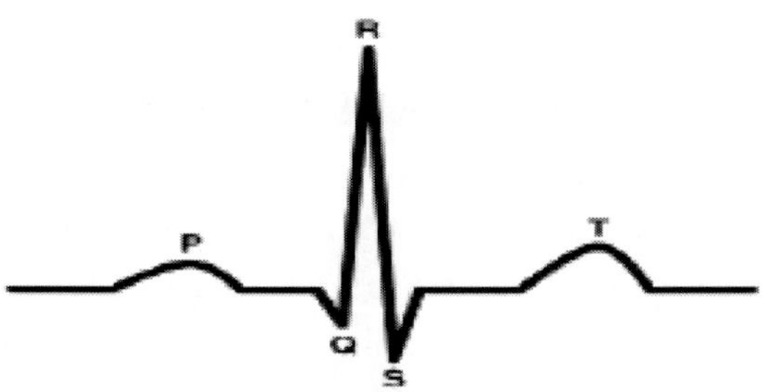

Figure 1.2. A typical cardiac cycle.

Each ECG wave in a cardiac cycle represents a physiological activity of the heart. The cycle of the electrical activity of the heart starts with the P wave, typically of less than 110ms duration represents atrial depolarization (contraction). Some abnormalities related to the atria, including left/right atrial hypertrophy and atrial premature beat can be detected from the P wave. There is a horizontal line segment at the isoelectric level between the P wave and the Q wave; this is the PQ (or PR when Q is absent) interval. Typically, the PQ interval is about 120-200ms duration. Some of the heart diseases may cause a shorter or longer PR interval. Next to the PQ wave in the graph is QRS complex, which is with a sharp peak at middle, called an R wave. The QRS complex represents the ventricular depolarization which may be typically about 60-100ms duration. In fact, the atrial depolarization (deactivation) occurs during the same interval, but it is not noticeable. Many ailments like cardiac arrhythmias, myocardial infarction, conduction abnormalities can be detected from the QRS complex. Since the QRS complex is the most dominant feature of the ECG cycle, it is used for determining the heart rate for a normal cardiac rhythm. The next important wave representing the ventricular repolarization is called T wave. The interval between the start of QRS complex and the peak of the T wave is called an absolute refractory period. The segment between the end of the QRS complex and the beginning of the T wave is called the ST segment, which lies at the same level as PQ segment. ST segment has a normal duration of 80-120ms. ST and T waves are analyzed for detection of myocardial infarction and ischemia. For a normal functioning heart, the cardiac cycle repeats continuously in the same ordered manner and time of repetition of the cardiac cycle determines the heart rate, which is variable due to many different physiological aspects, for example respiration rate, physical stress, anxiety, etc. [122]. This ECG signal comprising of the different waves are collected by the Ag/Agcl electrodes by placing on the body surface. These signals are within the frequency range of 0.05 to 100 Hertz (Hz.) or cycles per second. For accurate diagnosis clean, high resolution ECG signals have to be extracted from signals masked by various artifacts to ensure various parameters mentioned above. Therefore, it is important to develop noise cancellers to remove artifacts, so as to facilitate better diagnosis [184, 187].

1.3.1. Artifacts Due to Physiological Effects

One of the pre-requisites for obtaining a good ECG signal is for the subject to remain relaxed and still with no movements. Coughing, tensing of muscles and movement of the limbs causes the corresponding undesired artifacts in the ECG signal. In the absence of any movement of the subject, the only muscular activity in the body would be that of the heart. In [101] R. M. Raggayyan mentioned that dominant artefacts due to physiological reasons are Muscle Artefacts and Baseline Wandering.

1.3.1.1. Muscle Artifacts (MA)

Any muscular activity in the body produces a bio-potential signal which is also known as muscle artifacts. In recorded ECG, MA interference appears as rapid fluctuations which vary faster than ECG waves. In 1991 N. V. Tagore et al. [12] observed that MA noise in the ECG can be detected by measuring degree of signal fluctuation excluding the fluctuations of QRS complex. The peak amplitude of the MA signal on the surface of the body is in the range from 0.1 to 1mV and the spectrum is concentrated on the frequency range from 5 to 500Hz. Since the MA and ECG signals have partly overlapping spectra, the muscular activity may cause interference in the ECG signal. This type of noise can be reduced by making the patient comfort i.e., patient in a rest condition; this is suitable for short time monitoring. However, for long term monitoring under ambulatory condition high frequency MA noise is problematic and must be filtered out [19]. Figure 1.3 shows an ECG signal corrupted by MA noise.

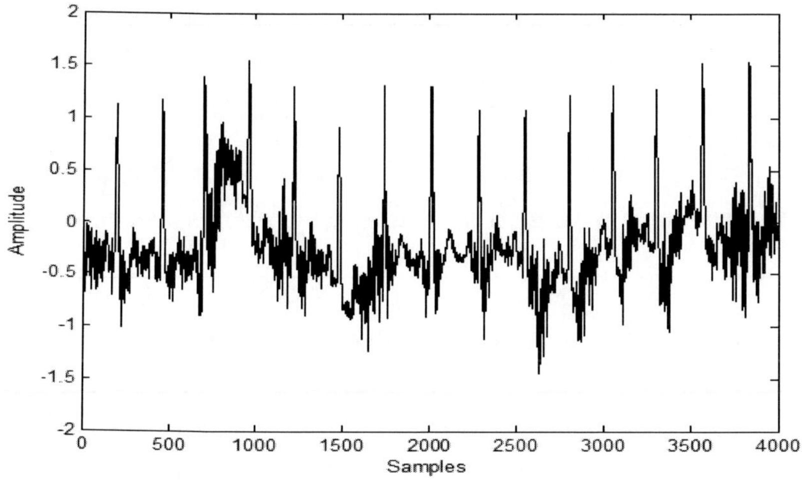

Figure 1.3. ECG signal corrupted with muscle artifacts.

1.3.1.2. Baseline Wander (BW)

The baseline of the ECG should ideally be at a constant level referred to as the isoelectric level. However, variations in lung volume due to respiration alter the path impedance between the ECG electrodes, causing a slowly varying potential difference for a constant current. Omid Sayadi et al. [24] defining baseline wander is a low-frequency noise (below 1Hz) resulting from respiration, reported that it occupies the same frequency band as the ST segment of the ECG signal. When chest leads are used,

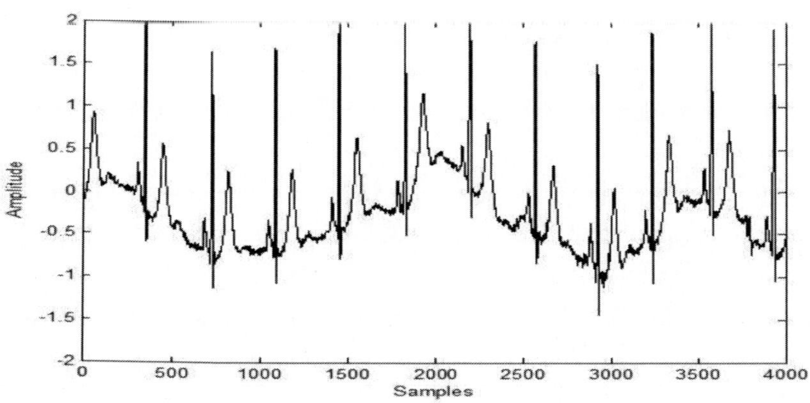

Figure 1.4. ECG signal corrupted with baseline wandering.

even normal breathing can cause the associated EMG of the chest muscles to interfere with desired ECG. According to N. V. Takore et al. [12] breathing causes beat to beat variations in the R-R interval, which should not be mistaken for sinus arrhythmia. Precision measurement of the ST segment depends on the effective removal of the baseline wander. Figure 1.4 shows the shift in the ECG signal caused by baseline wander.

1.3.2. Artifacts Due to Non-Physiological Effects

Apart from physiological artifacts, due to non-physiological reasons also ECG signal gets corrupted. The major non-physiological artifacts occurred in cardiac signals are Power Line Interference and Electrode Motion Artifacts [101].

1.3.2.1. Power Line Interference (PLI)

Power line interference coupled to signal carrying cables is particularly troublesome in medical equipment such as electrocardiograms. In 1975 B. Windrow et al. [13] observed that the cables carrying ECG signals from the examination room to the monitoring equipment are susceptible to electromagnetic interference (EMI) of power frequency (50 Hz or 60 Hz) by ubiquitous supply lines and plugs so much so that sometimes the ECG signal is totally masked by this type of noise. Filtering such EMI signal is a challenging problem given that the frequency of the time-varying power line signal lies within the frequency range of the ECG signal. 60Hz power line noise can affect the Q and P-waves of the ECG signal, generating errors during the diagnosis of arrhythmia. Power line noise can cause errors by distorting the ECG signal during the measurement of the QRS complex interval or the QT interval, which are important parameters in the diagnosis. The effect of PLI is shown in Figure 1.5. PLI masks the tiny features of the ECG signal and must be removed to enable accurate, through diagnosis. In 2008 Y. Der Lin et al. [25] presented an adaptive technique to detect and suppress PLI.

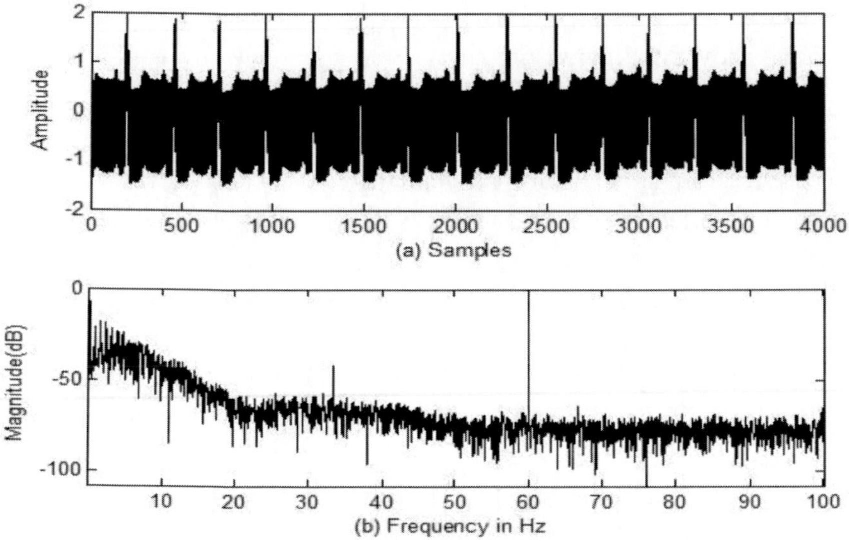

Figure 1.5. (a). ECG signal corrupted with PLI, (b). Spectrum of ECG signal with PLI.

1.3.2.2. Electrode Motion Artifacts (EM)

As the name suggests, these artifacts are caused by the movement of the electrodes against the skin. The electrical contact between the skin and the lead cable can be modelled as a network of equivalent resistors and capacitors representing the electrical parameters of different layers of the skin and the skin electrode interface.

The values of these electrical parameters may be altered due to relative motion of the electrodes or skin stretch or contract. This means that the equivalent impedance of the skin and the skin electrode interface gets disturbed due to any such action which results in an artifact known as motion artifact. Unfortunately, the motion artifact has a significant overlap with the spectrum of the ECG signal in the frequency range 1-10 Hz and hence it is very difficult to handle this type of artifact. It is noted that the motion artifact is more abrupt and distinct in nature as opposed to the slow baseline wander caused due to respiration. Reduction of motion interference for ECG measurements is desirable in many clinical and research situations, including long term ECG monitoring as well as ambulatory and exercise ECGs. An ECG signal corrupted by motion artifact is shown in Figure 1.6.

In 2005 M. Izzetoglu et al. [38] reported that the motion artifact was the most difficult form of the noise to be eliminated from ECG signals. This is because its spectrum completely overlaps that of the ECG, its morphology often resembles that of P, QRS and T waves. The motion artifacts were considered to be lower than 5Hz sinusoidal wave and filtered using over sampled (2KHz) ECG signal for better timing resolution.

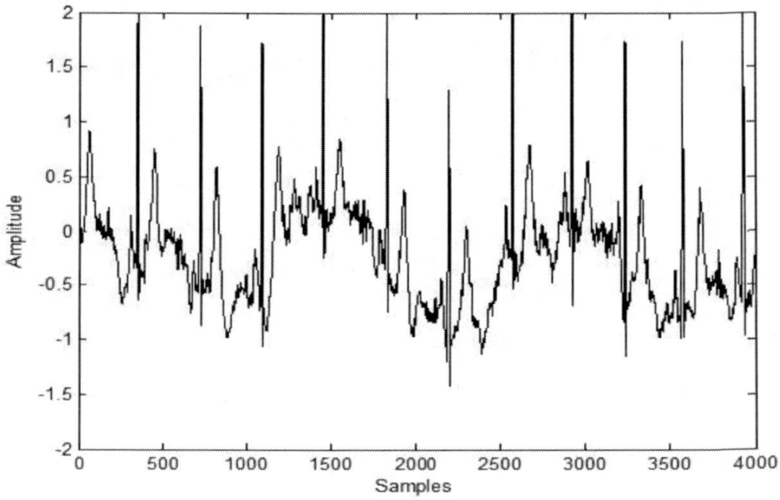

Figure 1.6. ECG signal corrupted with electrode motion artifacts.

1.4. Problem Definition

The ECG signal includes numerous artifacts, created during acquisition and transmission. The origins and nature of these artifacts are of considerable interest, particularly for long-term monitoring applications. As well as artifacts of both physiological and non-physiological origins, biotelemetry signals are affected by random channel noise. R. M. Rangayyan [101] points out that the presence of artifacts will make any morphology-based diagnosis problematic. In practice, most of the signals are non-stationary and any effective filter would have to be adaptive, adjusting its coefficients efficiently in accordance with the statistical nature of the noisy input signal. The development of efficient adaptive noise cancellers to remove artifacts from ECG signals would therefore be very beneficial.

The computational complexity of the adaptive filter in the receiver chain must be minimized, and complexity reduction of the noise cancellation technology in applications such as wireless biotelemetry systems has been a topic of intense research. It is vital work, as an increase in ECG data transmission rate increases the receiver impulse response length and thus the order of the filter. The resulting increase in complexity makes real time operation of the biotelemetry system difficult, especially in view of simultaneous shortening of the symbol period, which means that lesser time will be available to carry out the computations while the volume of the computations increasing.

Thus far, with reference to the literature, less attempts have been made to reduce the computational complexity of the adaptive noise canceller for denoising ECG signal without affecting the signal quality [44, 48, 72, 73]. To cope with both the complexity and convergence issues without any restrictive trade-off, we develop various adaptive filter structures to remove artifacts from the ECG signals on an embedded platform. This work builds on techniques and methods presented by [12] and proposes several efficient realizations. The next section outlines the contributions made in this regard.

1.5. A Review of Literature on ECG Enhancement

The development of ways to extract high-resolution ECG signals from recordings contaminated with background noise is an important issue. The goal of ECG signal enhancement is to separate the valid signal components from unwanted artifacts, thus facilitating easy and accurate interpretation of ECGs. The problem is a long-standing one and the literature is rich, so it is not possible to cover all the existing methods in detail. Due to the complexity of the problem, many of the existing methods use a combination of approaches, some borrowed from other contexts.

Telecardiology is a special branch of biotelemetry in which ECG signals travel wirelessly between the patient and diagnosis center. Many recent developments have been reported in the literature and show that telecardiology has a significant importance in cardiac health monitoring research. R. F. Yazicioglu et al. [123] presented the design and implementation of an analogue signal processor for portable ECG monitoring systems that targets ECG signal monitoring for accurate cardiac rhythm and heart rate variability analysis. Tee Hui Teo et al. [124] proposed a single-chip solution for wireless sensor nodes in a wireless health monitoring system, enabling a low-cost, small-form-factor and high-performance device that provides high-quality ECG signal acquisition.

Kyungtae Kang et al. [125] proposed the IEEE 802.11 wireless LAN as a promising solution, among several candidates for wireless ECG monitoring. These LANs, already deployed in many hospitals, can provide ubiquitous connectivity and thus allow cardiology patients greater mobility. IEEE 802.11 WLAN technology is simple, flexible, and cost-effective, suitable for use as a ubiquitous communication environment in hospitals. It obviates some of the problems of wireless networks, whose high collision rate and the resulting requirement for frequent retransmissions can cause unpredictable delays and jitters in a wireless network, thus degrading the quality of real-time ECG signals and necessitating further signal enhancement.

Reza S. Dilmaghani et al. [68] presented a wireless sensor network structure to monitor patients with chronic diseases in their own homes through a remote monitoring system of physiological signals. Their design needs no PC, as the nodes of the network are installed in the patients' homes and connected through the Internet to a central node at the hospital.

Sang Joon Lee et al. [130] developed a real-time data compression and transmission algorithm for a periodic ECG signal between e-health terminals. Their algorithm can compress and transmit data in real time, serving as a bio-signal data transmission method for limited bandwidth communication between e-health devices. However, channel noise and artifacts added to the bio-signal during acquisition degrade the quality of the signal, so further filtering is needed to obtain high resolution signals. Chin-Teng Lin et al. [135] presented a wireless, ambulatory, real-time biotelemetry system to improve cardiovascular health care. This device is connected to a mobile real-time display platform and an alert signal is sent to the remote database server, accessible through an Internet browser, once an abnormal ECG is detected. The system can identify abnormal cardiac rhythm in real time, an important ability benefitting both patients and healthcare personnel. The proposed system also activates an emergency medical alarm system when problems occur.

Piotr Augustyniak in [137] addresses the principal issues of the ECG interpretation adaptively in a distributed surveillance network. The background of such adaptively is the innovative use of results from the automatic ECG analysis to the seamless remote modification of the interpreting software. Since the medical relevance of issues diagnostic data depends on the patient's status, the interpretation adaptively implies the flexibility of report content and frequency. The entire above is made significant attempts for the development of sophisticated telecardiology systems, leaving the further research for noise cancellation.

L. Hadzievski et al. [128] presented the problem of synthesizing a standard 12-lead ECG from the signals recorded from only three ECG leads. The system has two separate units: a stationary diagnostic/calibration center and a mobile ECG device with integrated electrodes. The patient, acting alone, attaches three special leads from the mobile ECG recorder, which sends the recorded data by mobile phone to the PC in the diagnostic center, where the standard 12-lead ECG is numerically reconstructed using the patient transformation matrix previously calculated during preliminary calibration. Dewar D. Finlay et al. [129] proposed a method to record high-quality ECGs with the three bipolar leads located in the pericardial region. P Raphisak et al. [132] presented a non-adaptive morphological filter to remove muscle noise. They manually set a threshold for the noise, and accepted only signals that exceeded it.

Thakor and Zhu [12] presented an adaptive recurrent filter to remove muscle noise using a Least Mean Square (LMS) algorithm, proposing it as a useful method to acquire the impulse response of the normal QRS complex. The primary input of the filter is the ECG signal to be analyzed, while the reference input is an impulse train coincident with the QRS complexes.

Van Alste et al. [3] proved the concept of baseline wander and power line interference cancellation by using an efficient finite impulse response filter with a reduced number of taps. They proposed linear phase filtering for noise removal, periodically defining the desired filter spectrum to reduce the number of computations involved in digital filtering-as the spectrum period is 50Hz, the spectrum can be realised with many fewer impulse response coefficients. This, in combination with the necessary impulse response symmetry, leads to a reduction in the number of multiplications. Note, however, that this filtering technique is non-adaptive, as the filter cannot adjust its coefficients in accordance with the input noisy signal.

O. Sayadi et al. [5] developed a technique involving extraction of the characteristic points of ECG signals with baseline drift using bionic wavelet transform. As the frequency of baseline wander is 0.5 Hz, the noise component can be extracted by adjusting the frequency. This technique is not feasible for filtering randomly varying muscle artifact and channel noise. In 2005, Jacek et al. [30] introduced non-linear filter banks for the suppression of noise in ECG signals. Linear filters have long impulse responses that interrupt analysis; they overcame this disadvantage for some noise, but did not demonstrate that they had done so for non-stationary artifacts like MA and electrode motion. Ali et al. [31] presented a method for noise reduction using both non-linear filter banks and the wavelet approach.

Yunfeng et al. [133] presented an unbiased, normalised adaptive noise cancellation system using a two-stage moving-average filter and an infinite impulse response comb filter for the removal of periodic noise. This system is computationally more complex than one using the LMS-based filter system. B. V. Manuel et al. [134] developed an ECG enhancement

method based on the empirical mode decomposition for processing non stationary signals. The signal is decomposed into a sum of intrinsic mode functions with decreasing frequency content, so that the desired frequency components can be eliminated. Boucheham et al. [136] suggested a method for baseline correction based on pattern recognition tools called dominant points, computed by the Douglas-Peucker curve simplification algorithm. The points include peak and baseline points, the discrimination of which yields piecewise linear estimation of baseline wander in two iterations. At each iteration, the current baseline wander is subtracted from the input signal according to the decomposition scheme.

Hemilton [20] compared the performance of adaptive and non-adaptive notch filters used to remove the single-frequency component present in PLI. The author concluded that the adaptive filter requires no multiplications, but that implementation of the non-adaptive filter requires two multiplications, and that performance will vary with the sampling rate. The paper also confirms that long transient response times can hinder the filter's ability to track changes in noise amplitude, but does not go on to develop adaptive filters for the removal of non-stationary artifacts.

A. K. Ziarani et al. [22] proposed a technique for the elimination of PLI from ECG signals using a filter capable of extracting a specified component of a signal and tracking its variations over time. Better performance is observed in terms of effective elimination of noise under conditions of varying PLI frequency, but non-stationary noise cancellation is impossible because of the random characteristics of the noise signal.

Suzanna et al. [23] proposed an adaptive canceller for the suppression of PLI in ECG recordings. It tracks the amplitude, phase and frequency of both the fundamental component and the harmonics of the PLI, using a second-order phase-locked loop (PLL) in the design to handle frequency deviations. An error filter reduces the gradient noise caused by the ECG signal and the baseline wander. Parameter-adaptation blocking further reduces the gradient noise in the presence of large-amplitude segments of the QRS complex.

Y. Dir Lin et al. [25] presented a PLI detection and suppression algorithm to pre-process the ECG signals. It can detect the presence of PLI in the ECG signal and then apply the suppression algorithm. Their PLI detector employs an optimal linear discriminate analysis algorithm to decide whether or not PLI is present, and suppression is performed with an efficient recursive least-squares (RLS) adaptive notch filter. Note, however, that the RLS algorithm is more complex than the LMS algorithm.

Georgy et al. [32] described a PLI subtraction technique. Using moving averaging, interference is cancelled in linearly-going ECG segments that have near-zero frequency content; the extracted samples are saved in a buffer and then subtracted from the remaining parts of the signals.

The last decade has seen the presentation of many techniques for artifact removal. Mihov et al. [37] addressed the effect of motion artifacts and electrode impedance, while D.A. Tong et al. [138] proposed a method of reducing motion artifacts using an LMS based adaptive filter. Shen Luo et al. [139] proposed an adaptive technique for the removal of brachial motion artifacts in the ECG using LMS and RLS algorithms—the rate of convergence of RLS is faster than that of the LMS, but at the cost of higher computational complexity.

M. Milanesi et al. [140] proposed two different approaches to eliminate motion artifacts. The first approach, to counter electrode motion artifacts, is to place an accelerometer on the electrode, using its output in an adaptive filtering system to remove the noise present in the ECG. The second approach is based on independent component analysis methods applied to multichannel ECG recordings; the authors implemented adaptive filters based on both LMS and RLS algorithms.

Thakor et al. [12] proposed an LMS-based adaptive recurrent filter for the removal of motion artifacts. It adapts filter coefficients, enabling the acquisition of the impulse response of the desired signal, so is useful in cancelling noise from signals that have a repetitive morphology.

Many more approaches that address ECG enhancement have been reported in the literature. Murty et al. [1] introduced homomorphic analysis for ECG signals. This technique concentrates on computation of complex cepstrum, phase unwrapping and linear phase component removal, thus making diagnosis more efficient and less ambiguous. This strategy was originally used in speech processing. The authors considered four typical ECG signals and deconvolved them into their minimum and maximum phase components through cepstral filtering, with a view to study the possibility of more efficient feature selection from the component signals for diagnostic purposes. The complex cepstra of the signals are linearly filtered to extract the noise-free ECG signal.

In 1973, James et al. [2] addressed the problem of interference in ECG signals. They presented several causes of interference and suggested remedying them at circuit level. They concluded that: magnetic induction can be avoided by twisting the leads and keeping them close to the patient; interference caused by displacement current can be prevented by arranging leads such that displacement current in one is greater than in the other; and unsymmetrical electrode placement relative to differential AC potentials on the body causes interference which can be reduced by moving the earthed electrode. This paper does not introduce any signal processing techniques.

Kotas [4] presented principal component analysis-based ECG enhancement, Zhang et al. [6] and Yong et al. [7] presented baseline cancellation, T wave and QRST complex detection in ECG signals. Shao et al. [8], Lai et al. [9] and Reza et al. [11] analyzed fetal ECG signals under various circumstances. Ibrahim et al. [10] presented a morphological approach to remove baseline wander. In 2008, Valentina et al. [34] presented an analysis of the fibrillatory frequency trend and investigated time-dependent spectral characteristics using a spectral profile technique. T. Y. Ji et al. [35] described an approach to eliminate baseline drift from ECG signals, based on empirical mode decomposition and mathematical morphology.

Mihov et al. [37] addressed the effect of motion artifacts and electrode impedance in ECG signals. In 2008, Izzetoglu et al. [38] described motion artifact reduction in near-infrared spectroscopy measurements using Wiener filtering and more recently presented, a comparison of motion artifact removal in near-infrared spectroscopy [40]. Lemay et al. [41] reported a novel ventricular cancellation in ECG, using average beat subtraction and a single-beat method to cancel ventricular involvement independently in each cardiac cycle. Related work on ventricular and atrial fibrillation are reported in [42]-[43] and [142]. In 2010, Langley et al. used principal component analysis on beat-to-beat changes in ECG signals [39].

Ismet Sahin et al. [126] presented a new ECG enhancement approach for fetal wave forms in 2010. The fundamental period contains information indicating the physiological condition of the fetus, including hypoxia and academia, and to extract it, the discrete Fourier transforms (DFTs) of the fetal ECG waveform and its circularly shifted forms are measured. The optimal cosine waveform is then used to estimate the fundamental period. Comparison of this method with the cepstrum and average magnitude difference function methods shows that the DFT-based approach achieves very accurate period estimation results for both simulated and real fetal EGC waveforms taken at different stages of the gestation under noisy conditions.

1.6. Overview of the Book

This chapter has concentrated on the research objective and ECG background theory, providing a review of related literature. The introduction outlined the problem before explaining the motivation for the research in the light of the importance of ECG monitoring and the need for biotelemetry. Having described the basic nature of ECG signals and the various artifacts, physiological and non-physiological, that degrade them, the problem was discussed in more detail. A description of earlier work to counter the artifacts followed.

The authorities forbid experiments on humans or animals for the purposes of academic research, but as our main aim is investigation of various signal-processing algorithms for real-time implementation, so we have not recorded signals from human or animals. The entire data was taken from the MIT-BIH database. The stakeholders are the research community dedicated to ECG and other biomedical signal processing.

Chapter 2 elaborates the motivation behind the theme of this book, major research activities in adaptive noise canceller complexity reduction, the need for this reduction, and early work aimed at achieving it. There is an outline of the principle of the adaptive filter, its properties, convergence rate, maladjustment, tracking and computational requirements. The familiar LMS algorithm is fully discussed, as it is the reference algorithm for analysis purposes, the proposed methods are compared with it. We introduce a basic adaptive filter structure for noise cancellation in ECG signals, using its novel filter structures are designed to remove diverse forms of noise. These include power line interference, baseline wander, muscle artifact and electrode motion artifacts. Adaptive filtering is particularly suitable for biomedical signal processing as it allows estimation of the underlying signal in the absence of a prior knowledge of the statistical nature of the signal or noise.

Chapter 3 investigates the ways to enhance the existing methods and thus achieve better performance. The chapter, first concentrate on adaptive filters that stem from the LMS algorithm, considering four algorithms: namely, leaky LMS, dead zone LMS, least mean fourth and median LMS. In biotelemetry, a computationally less complex adaptive filter is desirable at the receiving end, so we extend the filters with their sign-based realizations; these are known to be simpler than their LMS-based counterparts, requiring only half as many multipliers. Three different versions of the sign-based algorithms are considered for this purpose: the signed regressor algorithm (SRA), sign algorithm (SA) and sign-sign algorithm (SSA). Sign-based treatment of all gradient algorithms requires appropriate modifications in the weight update recursion. The three versions of the simplified sign algorithms are combined with the LMS-based algorithms results sign-based version of the particular algorithm: sign regressor LMS, sign LMS, sign-sign LMS and so on. Including the LMS algorithm, five algorithms are considered and their sign-based versions. That produces another fifteen algorithms, giving a total of twenty algorithms to be implemented for ECG denoising. Finally, we use all these combinations to develop various adaptive noise cancellers (ANCs) for testing with real ECG signals. To evaluate the performance of the ANCs, convergence characteristics of all implementations are plotted before the computational complexity and signal-to-noise ratio improvement (SNRI),

EMSE and M_{ad} are calculated and compared with the conventional LMS algorithm.

Chapter 4 extends the LMS algorithm approach, with its sign-based realizations, by introducing a normalisation factor, usually employed with LMS-type filters to improve convergence speed. Here we consider both data and error normalizations. The data normalisation version of LMS, known as the NLMS algorithm, normalizes the correlation between the error and the reference input by a factor equal to the squared norm of the reference input signal vector. The major advantage of this algorithm is that the step size can be chosen independently of the reference signal power and the number of filter coefficients. Extension of NLMS by combining sign algorithms results in NSRLMS, NSLMS and NSSLMS algorithms. NSRLMS are derived from the SRA, where the normalising factor for the SRA equals the sum of the absolute values of the input signal vector components. The presence of the normalizing factor means that the steady-state error does not depend on the reference input signal power.

Error, as well as data, can be used for normalisation. An error-normalised LMS algorithm is known as an error non-linear LMS (ENLMS) algorithm. It's time-varying step-size is inversely proportional to the squared norm of error vector rather than the input data vector as in the NLMS algorithm. The sign-based realizations result in ENSRLMS, ENSLMS and ENSSLMS algorithms, which we use to develop various ANCs for testing in different statistical conditions and comparison with the conventional LMS algorithm. This chapter considers data- and error-normalised algorithms, with three signed versions of each, so eight algorithms are used altogether.

Chapter 5 presents an efficient block-based ANC implementation, considering both overlapping and non-overlapping blocks. As the input sequence grows, the adaptive filter length has to be increased, making the filter computationally complex. Block processing of input data significantly reduces the computational burden of the adaptive filter. In block processing, the data are processed block by block rather than sample by sample. Considering non-overlapping blocks first, we developed an ANC based on a Block LMS (BLMS). Recognizing that the Fourier transform maps time-domain signals in the frequency domain, we see that it is possible to adapt the filter coefficients in the frequency domain. The BLMS implemented in this domain is known as a Fast BLMS (FLMS). To benefit from fast convergence, we have also developed ANCs by combining BLMS with NLMS and ENLMS individually. This results in BNLMS and BENLMS algorithms in the time domain, their frequency domain realizations are known as FBNLMS and FBENLMS algorithms. That gives us six algorithms for ECG enhancement in the non-overlapping class. Next, we apply the approach of overlapping block processing to the normalised algorithms discussed in Chapter 4, producing block-based (BB) NLMS, BBENLMS and their SRA, SA and SSA versions. This overlapping approach gives eight algorithms. Finally, various ANCs are developed and tested using MATLAB; performance evaluation is carried with reference to computational complexity and SNRI. In total, we have developed 42 adaptive noise cancellers for the removal of artifacts from ECG signals.

In Chapter 6 we demonstrate the concept of noise cancellation in ECG signals on a real time embedded processor, using those algorithms from the previous chapters that show both good filtering capability and less computational complexity. These are: Sign Regressor LMS, Sign Regressor Dead Zone LMS, Normalised Sign Regressor LMS, Error Normalised Sign Regressor LMS, Frequency domain Block Normalised LMS, Frequency domain Block Error Normalised LMS, Block based Normalised Sign Regressor LMS and Block based Error Normalised Sign Regressor LMS algorithm. In addition to these eight algorithms, the LMS algorithm is considered for implementation for standardization purposes. This implementation confirms that the developed ANCs are acceptable in real-time environments. All the algorithms are implemented on an embedded TI TMS320C6713 digital signal processor.

Chapter 7 concludes the work presented in this book by summing up the salient features of all the proposed schemes and highlighting the related issues. In the previous chapters we have developed 42 adaptive noise cancellers for the removal of PLI, BW, MA and EM artifacts from ECG signals. All were tested using MATLAB and 8 of them developed and tested on an embedded platform, the TI TMS320C6713 digital signal processor. To do this, eight algorithms, originally written in MATLAB, were rewritten in the C language for processor implementation. For standardization of the results, a conventional LMS based noise canceller was developed and compared with the newly-developed ANCs. Experimental results confirm that the developed noise cancellers are superior to the conventional LMS algorithm in ECG denoising applications.

Chapter 2

THEORETICAL CONSIDERATIONS OF ADAPTIVE FILTERING TECHNIQUES

2.1. INTRODUCTION

The term filter is commonly used to refer any device or system that takes a mixture of particles or elements from its input and process them according to some specific rules to generate a corresponding set of particles or elements in its output. More specifically, a filter can a system that reshapes the frequency components of the input to generate an output signal with some desirable features. Figure 2.1 depicts a general schematic diagram of such a filter emphasizing its role in reshaping the input signal to match the desired signal [86]. This chapter elaborates the important theory related to adaptive filtering, explaining the adaptive filter, its properties, the need for adaptive filtering in biotelemetry, the least mean square algorithm, the structure of adaptive noise canceller, the need for the development of new adaptive noise cancellers. There is also a review of the literature on adaptive signal processing and a conclusion.

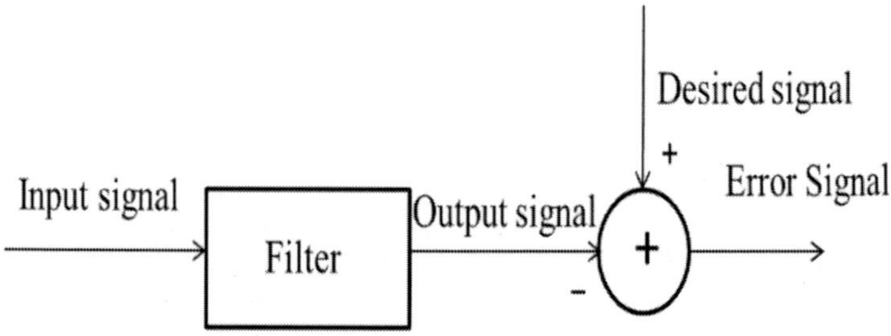

Figure 2.1. Basic schematic of a filter.

2.1.1. Adaptive Filter

In practical situations, most signals are non-stationary in nature, but the conventional filters like FIR, IIR and Notch, all have fixed filter coefficients and apply the same degree of signal conditioning irrespective of the degree of noise on the input signal. In such situations, these fixed coefficient, non-adaptive filters are not suitable. In order to filter time varying non-stationary components, the filter coefficients must vary in accordance with input signal characteristics. Adaptive filters have this capability, they are able to change their filter coefficients in accordance with input signal characteristics [100, 113].

2.1.2. Properties of Adaptive Algorithms

The basic operation of an adaptive filter is to minimize an objective function, generally denoted by J_w. By proper selection of this objective function one can condition it to have a continuous shape [100]. The choice of one algorithm over another is determined by one or more of the following factors.

1. *Rate of convergence:* This is defined as the number of iterations required for the algorithm, in response to stationary inputs, to converge "close enough" to the optimum wiener solution in the mean-square error sense. The convergence curve can be plotted by measuring mean square

error (MSE) at each iteration, and plotting the curve between and the number of iterations. The MSE is given by the relation,

$$\xi = E\{|e(n)|^2\} \tag{2.1}$$

where ξ is mean square error and e (n) is the error signal.

2. *Misadjustment:* For an algorithm of interest, this parameter provides a quantitative measure of the amount by which the final value of the mean-square error, averaged over an ensemble of adaptive filters, deviates from the minimum mean square error. This is formally defined as,

$$M_{ad} = \frac{EMSEss}{MMSE} \tag{2.2}$$

where $EMSE_{ss}$ is the steady state value of excess mean square error (EMSE), the MMSE is the minimum mean square error. Misadjustment is a dimension less parameter that provides a measure how close the algorithm is to optimality in the mean square error sense.

The MMSE is the optimum filtering error, which represents the portion of the primary signal that cannot be cancelled by the optimal weight. It can be defined by averaging out signal power over samples after which the algorithm reaches the steady state. This is given by

$$MMSE = \frac{1}{k-p}\sum_{n=p}^{k}|x(n)|^2 \tag{2.3}$$

Here k is the total number of the samples and p is the number of samples at which the algorithm reaches steady state. The EMSE caused by the deviation of the weights from their optimal values is defined as,

$$EMSE(n) = \frac{1}{N}\sum_{j=0}^{N-1}|e_1(n-j)| \tag{2.4}$$

where $e_l(n)$ are the residual error and N is the number of samples used in the estimation. The steady state EMSE is defined by taking the EMSE over a certain duration after the convergence characteristics is obtained.

$$EMSE_{ss} = \frac{1}{k-p} \sum_{n=P}^{K} EMSE(k) \tag{2.5}$$

3. *Tracking:* when an adaptive filtering algorithm operates in a non-stationary environment, the algorithm is required to track statistical variation in the environment. The tracking performance of the algorithm is influenced by two contradictory features: (1) rate of convergence (2) steady-state fluctuation due to algorithmic noise.

4. *Computational requirements:* Here the issues of concern include the number of operations required to make on complete iteration of the algorithm. Normally in signal processing applications the complexity of the algorithm is measured in terms of number of multiplications and accumulation (MAC) operations required to perform the operation. Between multiplication and addition, multiplication is complex. So, in complexity reduction techniques the number of multiplications has to be minimized.

2.2. Need of Adaptive Filtering in Biotelemetry

The ECG signal contains numerous artifacts that must be removed by a filter before monitoring to display an accurate signal. The FIR and IIR filters provide considerable flexibility in altering the frequency content of a signal. These filters can provide almost any desired frequency characteristic to nearly any degree of accuracy. The actual frequency characteristic attained by the various design routines can be verified through the Fourier Transform analysis. However, the design routines do not tell the user that which frequency characteristic is the best i.e., what type of filtering will most effectively separate out signal from noise. That decision is made based on the user's knowledge of signal or source properties. The optimal filter theory was developed to provide structure to the process of selecting the most appropriate frequency characteristic. If the representation of the desired signal is available, then a well-developed and popular class of filters known as wiener filter can be applied. The basic concept behind wiener filter theory is to minimize the mean square value of the error signal defined as the difference between the desired response and the actual filter output. A plot of the mean square value of the error signal versus the adjustable parameters of a linear filter is referred to as the error performance surface. The minimum point of this surface represents the Wiener solution. As the Wiener filter is inadequate for dealing with non-stationary signals, the optimum filter has to assume a time varying form when such signals are encountered. The Wiener filter requires a priori information about the statistics of the data to be processed, and remains optimum only as long as the statistical characteristics of the input data match the information on which the filter design is based. When this information is not known completely it may not be possible to design the Wiener filter, or else the design may no longer be optimum. So, we go for adaptive filter, such a system is self-designing which relies for its operation on a recursive algorithm which makes it possible for the filter to perform satisfactorily in an environment where the complete knowledge of the relevant signal characteristics is not available. The algorithm starts from some predetermined set of initial conditions, represents whatever we know about the environment. Yet in a stationary environment we find that after successive iterations of the algorithm it converges to optimum wiener solution in some statistical sense. In a non-stationary environment, the algorithm offers a tracking capability provided that the variations are sufficiently small [86].

In recent years, adaptive filtering has become an effective and popular approach for processing and analysis of ECG and other biomedical signals. Adaptive filters permit detection of time varying potentials and tracking the dynamic variations of the signals. They also modify their behavior according to the input signal. This means that they can detect shape variations in the ensemble and thus obtain a better signal estimation. Several papers have been presented in the area of biomedical signal processing where an adaptive solution based on the LMS algorithm is suggested [12, 26].

2.3. THE LEAST MEAN SQUARE (LMS) ALGORITHM

The LMS algorithm is a linear adaptive filtering algorithm that consists of two processes.

1. *Filtering Process:* Computing the output of the transversal filter produced by a set of inputs and generating an estimation error by comparing this output to a desired response.
2. *An adaptive process:* This involves automatic adjustment of the tap weights of the filter in accordance with the estimation error [96], [100].

In adaptive filter, usually a transversal filter structure is employed shown in the Figure 2.1. Let the input to the filter n_2 be assigned as **x(n)**. The tap inputs x(n), x(n – 1), x(n – 2), ... x(n – L + 1) forms the elements of the L-by-1 tap input vector **x(n)**, where L-1 are the number of delay elements. Correspondingly, the tap weights $\mathbf{w(n)} = [w_0, w_1, \dots, w_{L-1}]^T$ form the elements of the L-by-1 tap-weight vector w. The value computed for this vector using the LMS algorithm represents an estimate whose expected value may come close to the wiener solution w_0 as the number of iterations *n*, approaches infinity [86].

The output of the FIR filter is the inner product of **x(n)** and **w(n)**

$$y(n) = \mathbf{x}(\boldsymbol{n})^{\mathrm{T}}\,\mathbf{w(n)} = \mathbf{w(n)}^{T}\,\mathbf{x}(\boldsymbol{n}) \tag{2.6}$$

The error $e(n)$ is defined as the difference between the desired response $d(n)$ and the actual response $y(n)$.

$$e(n) = d(n) - y(n) \tag{2.7}$$

The mean square error is given as

$$\xi = E\{|e(n)|^2\} = E\{|d(n) - y(n)|^2\} \tag{2.8}$$

The LMS adaptive algorithm is a practical method for finding a close approximate solution to the above one in real time. The algorithm does not require explicit measurements of correlation functions, nor does it involve matrix inversion. Accuracy is limited by statistical sample size. The LMS algorithm is an implementation of the method of steepest descent. According to this method, the next weight vector **w(n + 1)**, is equal to the present weight vector **w(n)** plus a change proportional to the negative gradient:

$$\boldsymbol{w(n+1)} = \boldsymbol{w(n)} - \mu\nabla\xi(n) \tag{2.9}$$

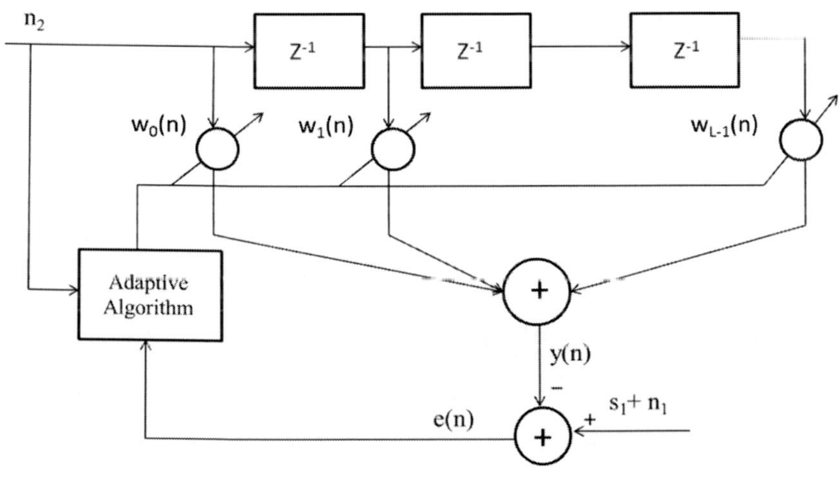

Figure 2.2. Transversal filter.

The step size μ affects the rate at which the weight vector moves down the quadratic surface and must be a positive number (a negative value of μ would move the weight vector up the quadratic surface in the direction of maximum ascent and would result in an increase in error). For the small value of step size μ the correction applied to the **w** ***(n)*** is small and the movement down the quadratic surface is slow and as the step size parameter μ has increased the rate of decent increase. However, there is an upper limit on how large the step size may be, for a value μ exceeds this limit, the trajectory of $\mathbf{w}(\boldsymbol{n})$ becomes unstable and unbounded [96]. However, the recursive computation of each tap weight in the LMS algorithm suffers from a gradient noise [100].

Where

$$\nabla\xi(n) = \nabla E\{|e(n)|^2\} = E\{\nabla|e(n)|^2\} = E\{e(n)\nabla e^*(n)\} \quad (2.10)$$

and $\nabla e^*(n) = -\boldsymbol{x}^*(\boldsymbol{n})$

(2.11)

Substituting (2.11) in (2.10) results

$$\nabla\xi(n) = -E\{e(n)\boldsymbol{x}^*(\boldsymbol{n})\} \quad (2.12)$$

Now substituting (2.12) in (2.9)

$$w(n+1) = w(n) + \mu E\{e(n)\boldsymbol{x}^*(\boldsymbol{n})\} \quad (2.13)$$

A practical limitation with this algorithm is that Expectation $E\{e(n)\boldsymbol{x}^*(\boldsymbol{n})\}$ is generally unknown. Therefore, it must be replaced with an estimate such as the sample mean

$$\hat{E}\{e(n)\boldsymbol{x}^*(\boldsymbol{n})\} = \frac{1}{L}\sum_{l=0}^{L-1} e(n-l)\,\boldsymbol{x}^*(\boldsymbol{n}-\boldsymbol{l}) \quad (2.14)$$

Incorporating this estimation into the steepest decent

$$\boldsymbol{w}(\boldsymbol{n}+\mathbf{1}) = \boldsymbol{w}(\boldsymbol{n}) + \mu\frac{1}{L}\sum_{l=0}^{L-1} e(n-l)\,\boldsymbol{x}^*(\boldsymbol{n}-\boldsymbol{l}) \quad (2.15)$$

In LMS we use 1-pt sample mean $L = 1$ such that

$$\hat{E}\{e(n)\boldsymbol{x}^*(\boldsymbol{n})\} = e(n)\boldsymbol{x}^*(\boldsymbol{n}) \qquad (2.16)$$

In this case the weight update equation becomes

$$w(n + 1) = w(n) + \mu e(n)\boldsymbol{x}^*(\boldsymbol{n}) \qquad (2.17)$$

and it is known as LMS algorithm. This algorithm will converge in the mean and will remain stable as long as the parameter μ is greater than 0 but less than twice the reciprocal of the largest eigen value λ_{max}, of the input autocorrelation matrix R_x.

$$0 < \mu < \frac{2}{\lambda_{max}}$$

The problem with LMS algorithm is that selecting the step size parameter μ, smaller the value of μ convergence will be slow but the steady state error will be small. On the other hand, larger the value of μ convergence will be fast, but the steady state error will be more. So, selecting the proper value of μ is difficult in LMS algorithm. Another problem is step size parameter μ is dependent on the input signal power and moreover as the weight vector begins to converge in the mean, the coefficients begin to fluctuate about their optimum values. These fluctuations are due to the noisy gradient vectors that are used to form the corrections to w(n). As a result, the variance of the weight error vector does not go to zero and the mean-square error is larger than the minimum mean-square error by an amount referred to as the excess mean-square error. That is the convergence analysis of the LMS algorithm with deterministic reference inputs showed that the steady-state weight vector is biased.

2.4. THE STRUCTURE OF AN ADAPTIVE NOISE CANCELLER TO REMOVE ARTIFACTS FROM ECG SIGNALS

The structure of an adaptive noise canceller is shown in Figure 2.3. Let the transmitted ECG signal be 's_1' transmitted over a channel to a sensor that also receives a noise n_1 uncorrelated with the signal. The combined signal and noise $s_1 + n_1$ form the primary input to the canceller. A second sensor receives a noise n_2 uncorrelated with the signal, but correlated in some unknown way with the noise n_1. This sensor provides the reference input to the canceller. The noise n_2 is filtered to produce an output y that is as close as possible, a replica of n_1. This output is subtracted from the primary input $s_1 + n_1$ to produce the system output $e = s_1 + n_1 - y$. If one knew the characteristics of the channels over which the noise was transmitted to the primary and reference sensors, it would theoretically be possible to design a fixed filter capable of changing n_2 into n_1. The filter output could then be subtracted from the primary input, and the system output would be signal alone. Since the characteristics of the transmission paths are unknown (or known only approximately) and are seldom of a fixed nature, the use of a fixed filter is not feasible. Even if it were, its characteristics would have to be adjusted with a precision difficult to attain, and the slightest error could result in an increase in output noise power. In the system shown in Figure 2.4 the reference input is processed by an adaptive filter unlike a fixed filter automatically adjusts its own impulse response [12].

Adjustment is accomplished through an algorithm that responds to an error signal dependent, among other things, on the filter's output. Thus, with the proper algorithm, the filter can operate under changing conditions and can readjust itself continuously to minimize the error signal. The error signal used in an adaptive process depends on the nature of the application. In noise cancelling systems the practical objective is to produce a system output $e = s_1 + n_1 - y$ that is a best fit in the least squares sense to the signal s_1. This objective is accomplished by feeding the system output back to the adaptive filter and adjusting the filter through adaptive algorithms to minimize total system output power.

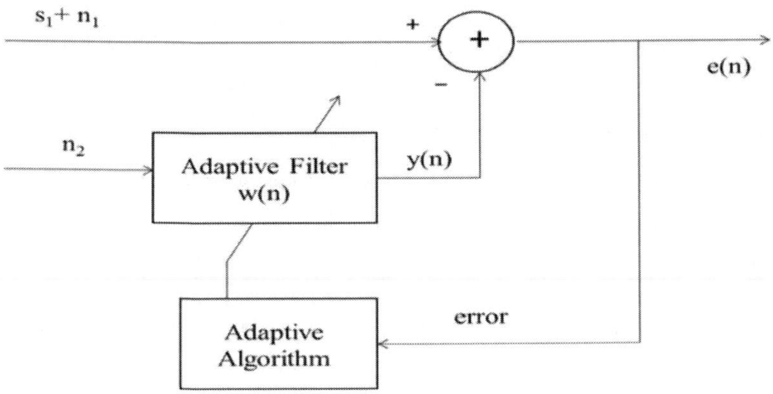

Figure 2.3. Structure of an adaptive noise canceller.

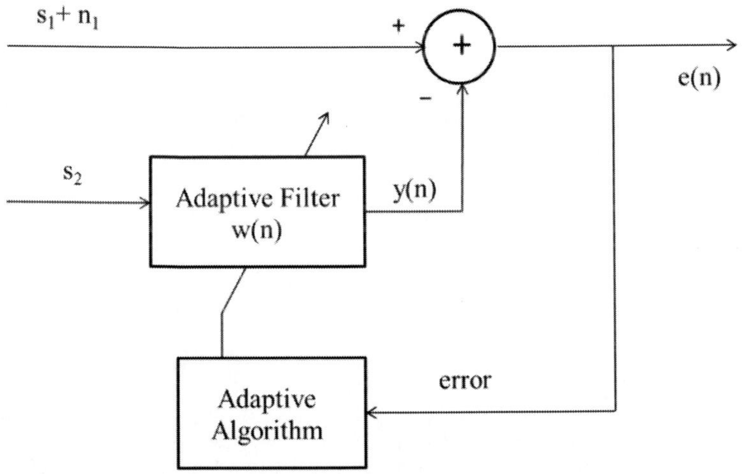

Figure 2.4. An alternative structure of adaptive noise canceller.

In an adaptive noise cancelling system, in other words, the system output serves as the error signal for the adaptation process. Now assume that s_1, n_1, n_2, and y are statistically stationary and have zero means. Assume also that s_1 is uncorrelated with n_1 and n_2, and suppose that n_2 is correlated with n_1. The output e is given as

$$e = s_1 + n_1 - y \tag{2.18}$$

Squaring on both sides results

$$e^2 = s_1^2 + (n_1 - y)^2 + 2s_1(n_1 - y) \tag{2.19}$$

Taking Expectation on both sides to the above equation and realizing that s_1 is uncorrelated with n_1 and with y, yields

$$E[e^2] = E[s_1^2] + E[(n_1 - y)^2] + 2E[s_1(n_1 - y)] \tag{2.20}$$

$$= E[s_1^2] + E[(n_1 - y)^2] \tag{2.21}$$

The signal power $E[s_1^2]$ will be unaffected as the filter is adjusted to minimize $E\,[e^2]$.

Accordingly, the minimum output power is

$$min\,E[e^2] = minE[s_1^2] + minE[(n_1 - y)^2] \tag{2.22}$$

When the filter is adjusted so that $E\,[e^2]$ is minimized, $E\,[(n_1 - y)^2]$ is, therefore, also minimized. The filter output y is then a best least square estimate of the primary noise n_1. Moreover, when E $[(n_1 - y)^2]$ is minimized, $E[(e - s_1)^2]$ is also minimized, since, from the (2.18) we have,

$$(e - s_1) = (n_1 - y) \tag{2.23}$$

Adjusting or adapting the filter to minimize the total output power cause the output e to be a best least square estimate of the signal s_1 for the given structure and adjustability of the adaptive filter and for the given reference input. The output e will contain the signal $E\,[e^2]$ plus noise. From (2.18), the output noise is given by (n_1 – y). Since minimizing $E[e^2]$ minimizes $E[(n_1 - y)^2]$, minimizing the total output power minimizes the output noise power. Since the signal in the output remains constant, minimizing the total output power maximizes the output signal-to- noise ratio. It is seen that from the above equation that the smallest possible output power is $E[e^2] = E[s_1^2]$. This is achievable when $E[(n_1 - y)^2] = 0$. Therefore, $y = n_1$, and $e = s_1$. In this case, minimizing output power causes the output signal to be perfectly noise free. As we can see from the above adaptive filter structure the error signal e is fed back to the adaptive algorithm, and depending upon this algorithm the filter weight adjusts to the changing environment.

Figure 2.4 illustrates another situation where the ECG is recorded from several electrode leads [12]. The primary input $s_1 + n_1$ is a signal from one the leads. A reference signal s_2 is obtained from a second lead that is noise free. The signal s_1 can be extracted by minimizing the MSE between the primary and the reference inputs. Generally, in biomedical signal processing, the filter structure shown in Figure 2.4 is generally used, since it is difficult to obtain a noise free signal. Using the same procedure similar to (2.19) we can show that,

$$E[e^2] = E[(s_1 - y)^2] + E[n_1^2] \tag{2.24}$$

Minimizing the MSE results in a filter error output y that is the best least-squares estimate of the signal s_1.

2.5. Need for the Development of New Adaptive Noise Cancellers

In biomedical signal processing the statistical nature of the signal varies from sample to sample [101]. In such case the filter which we are using for the development of noise canceller must be able to change its filtering coefficients from sample to sample depending on signal levels [163]. Adaptive filter has this ability, since no or almost no prior information is available, an adaptive filter requires an initial period for learning or adaptation. During this period, its performance is unsatisfactory; as a result, the convergence rate is slow at the initial stage.

The fundamental adaptive algorithm, least mean square (LMS) algorithm suffers from two problems. First, when the input data vector is large, LMS algorithm suffers a gradient noise amplification problem [100]. Secondly, its convergence rate is slow because of its fixed step size. Computational complexity is also large, SNR is limited, it is sensitive to round off errors and liable to weight drift. In clinical situations, these drawbacks have to be avoided [96].

To overcome these problems, we propose the development of various adaptive noise cancellers (ANCs) using different categories of adaptive algorithms. The objective of the new ANCs for ECG enhancement is fast convergence, low computational complexity and. In order to achieve this, we classify the adaptive algorithms in three categories,

1. Weight update variants of LMS algorithm
2. Normalized adaptive algorithms
3. Block adaptive algorithms

In the first category, we consider weight update variants of the LMS algorithm, which can be directly derived from it. These are Leaky LMS (to avoid weight drift) [76], Dead Zone LMS (to diminish round off error) [160], Least mean fourth (to obtain a lower steady state error) [108] and Median LMS (to smooth the impulsive noise) [91]. To reduce the computational complexity, simplified algorithms are also combined with these algorithms [86]. These are sign regressor, sign and sign-sign algorithms.

In the second category, we introduce normalization. S. C. Douglas et al. [94] proved that normalisation makes the step size variable, giving fast convergence and good filtering capability. Here we use both data normalisation and error normalisation, giving two algorithms, Normalized LMS (NLMS) and Error-normalized LMS or error non-linear LMS (ENLMS) respectively. The advantage of ENLMS is that step size can be chosen independently of the input data value and number of tap weights [115]. Biotelemetry, however, demands low computational complexity of the adaptive filter as well as fast convergence and good filtering capability.

To achieve this, we combine NLMS and ENLMS algorithms with three simplified algorithms [99], giving us the normalized sign regressor (NSRLMS), normalized sign LMS (NSLMS), normalized sign-sign LMS (NSSLMS), error non-linear sign regressor LMS (ENSRLMS), error non-linear sign LMS (ENSLMS) and error non-linear sign-sign LMS (ENSSLMS) algorithms.

In the clinical environment, if the ECG signal to be processed contains a large number of samples, then sample-by-sample filtering causes large computational complexity. In such situations block processing is a better choice, and the third category in this research focuses on block-processing algorithms. The input signal is split into blocks containing a fixed number of samples and each block filtered separately and in order, a process known as non-overlapping block processing. The resulting algorithm is the Block LMS (BLMS) [102]. Implemented in the frequency domain to increase signal resolution, it is called a Fast BLMS (FBLMS), since it uses Fast Fourier Transform (FFT) to transform from time domain to frequency domain [104]. To increase the convergence rate and filtering capability, we introduce normalization with BLMS and FBLMS algorithms. We now have block normalized LMS (BNLMS), fast block normalized LMS (FBNLMS), block error non-linear LMS (BENLMS) and fast block error non-linear LMS (FBENLMS) algorithms. Overlapping block processing, a special case of NLMS and ENLMS algorithms, is also available. The input data is processed sample by sample, but the normalization is done block wise. We normalize the algorithm with respect to the maximum value of data values or error values in that particular iteration. The algorithms, thus created are the block-based NLMS (BBNLMS), block-based ENLMS (BBENLMS) and their simplified versions [107]. In this manner, variants and extensions of the original LMS algorithm result in a fast convergence rate, good filtering capability (high SNR) and low computational complexity, all useful characteristics for ECG enhancement in biotelemetry applications.

2.6. Review of Literature on Adaptive Signal Processing

With the rapid growth of adaptive signal processing, many contributions are appearing in the literature; some are mentioned here. Ali et al. [49] proposed a method that indicates how close the adaptive filter is to optimal performance. Using this, the authors developed a variable step-size affine projection algorithm and a variable step-size NLMS (VSSNLMS) algorithm. The simulation results confirm that these exhibit a faster convergence rate and lower misadjustment error.

Similarly, Vega et al. [50] presented a framework for a robust VSSNLMS algorithm based on optimization of cost function subject to a time-dependent constraint on the norm of the filter update. The authors have tested this in identification and echo cancellation applications.

Another VSSNLMS for acoustic echo cancellation is reported by Paleologu et al. [51]. The authors noted that previously implemented algorithms dealt with exact modelling simulations, where the length of the adaptive filter equals the length of the system to be modelled. In practice, the acoustic echo paths are extremely long, so it would be beneficial if the filter were shorter than the path. They then went on to use that strategy in their solution.

Ching Lai [52] presented an NLMS-based IIR filter. This method proved that an LMS-SAS (stochastic approximation with convolution smoothing) algorithm is better than GLMS in global optimization terms, and that NLMS is better than LMS-SAS. The author also declared that a decrease in step size in NLMS does not play the crucial role that it does in GLMS.

Ahmed et al. [53] analyzed the convergence and steady state analysis of a VSSNLMS algorithm. This algorithm eliminates the trade-off between residue error and convergence speed. Several types of VSSLMS algorithms are presented in [54, 55, 64]. Mean square error (MSE) is the key element in adaptive filtering.

Y. N. Rao et al. [56] presented a new argument on MSE, the error whitening criterion (EWC). This criterion is capable of eliminating bias when noise is white. The authors developed some stochastic gradient and fast algorithms to measure the EWC solution online. The structures and complexity of these algorithms are similar to those of LMS and NLMS. This can also discussed a recursive least square-like recursive error whitening (REW) algorithm and a minor component analysis-based EWC total least squares algorithm. They assessed the noise rejection capability of EWC by comparing its performance with that of the MSE criterion and total least squares.

The major drawback of the familiar LMS algorithm is that it is a compromise between speed of convergence and final misadjustment. To overcome this problem, Arenas et al. [57] used a combination of two LMS filters. The concept of combinational LMS is extended in two directions. The first is a combined multiple LMS filter with different steps, and the second is a different mixing parameter for each weight of the filter in order to make their adaptation speed independent. However, the computational complexity of the new algorithms increases with the number of filters and their tap length.

The correlated input sequence tends to degrade in convergence characteristics in an LMS filter. An affine projection algorithm (APA) can be used to overcome this. Its main purpose is to speed up the convergence, particularly in correlated sequences, but computational complexity is a weak point in the APA implementation. Hwang et al. [58] presented an APA with reduced complexity by selecting a subset of input regressors at each iteration. The finest choice of input regressors is obtained by comparing cost functions based on the principle of minimum disturbance. This technique shows better performance of the algorithm in simulations.

Weissman et al. [59] proposed a universal filter whose per symbol squared error is essentially smaller than the best FIR filter of the same order. Instead of updating all tap weights at every iteration, a subset of weight coefficients is updated at every iteration on criteria that depend on energy conservation of the input sequence. The mean square performance of such partial update filter is presented in [60] by Abadi et al. The convergence rate of NLMS can be improved by a normalised sub-band adaptive filter (NSAF).

J Ni et al. [61] proposed a VSSNSAF to recover the powers of the sub-band system noises from the sub-band error signals of the adaptive filter. Simulation results show that maladjustment is low and performance of the algorithm better than that of the other NSAF algorithms. Like partial update filters, a proportionate NLMS (PNLMS) updates tap coefficients individually instead of globally, as in Souza's LMS [62]. Each individual activation factor is computed in terms of past and current values of the corresponding coefficient magnitude. That means that each activation factor presents some inherent memory associated with its corresponding coefficient magnitude. This strategy leads to a better allocation of adaptation energy over the tap weights than the conventional LMS does. Regalia et al. developed a complex adaptive notch filter to track single-sided tones immersed in background noise [63]. Although these contributions focused on the signal processing aspects of adaptive filters, none concentrated on the reduction of computational complexity desirable in biotelemetry applications.

In addition to these signal-conditioning contributions, several papers are presented in the context of ECG enhancement using adaptive filtering techniques. Thakor and Zhu [12] proposed an adaptive recurrent filter to acquire the impulse response of normal QRS complexes, and then applied it to arrhythmia detection in ambulatory ECG recordings. In this paper, different filter structures are presented to eliminate the diverse forms of noise: baseline wander, 60Hz power line interference, muscle noise and motion artefacts. An adaptive recurrent filter structure is proposed for acquiring the impulse response of the normal QRS complex. The primary input of the filter is the ECG signal to be analysed, while the reference input is an impulse train coincident with the QRS complexes. This method is applied to several arrhythmia detection problems: detection of P waves, premature ventricular complexes, and recognition of conduction block, atrial fibrillation and paced rhythm.

The fundamental principles of adaptive filtering for noise cancellation were described by I. Widrow [13], who presented the concept of adaptive noise cancellation to replace the direct subtraction of noise from signal. This is a dangerous procedure, if done improperly causes output noise power to rise. In this paper, the authors proposed several applications of adaptive cancellation, including cancellation of 60Hz interference in ECG signals, cancelling the donor ECG after heart transplantation, removing the maternal ECG from foetal ECGs, cancelling noise in speech signals and cancelling antenna side-lobe interference. They presented the analysis of an adaptive filter with two weights, using the LMS) algorithm. This paper gives a fundamental idea of noise cancellation with adaptive filtering, and Widrow et al. [13] and Thakor et al. [12] have made major contributions to the design of adaptive noise cancellers (ANC) for ECG enhancement.

Mark et al. [14] proposed to eliminate electrosurgical interference using radio frequency shielding, low pass filtering and optical isolation. Their aim was to use a combination of adaptive noise cancelling and conventional signal processing to enhance electrocardiographic monitoring in the operating room by reducing the noise interference created by an electrosurgical instrument. Their technique does remove significant amounts of interference. A digital adaptive canceller, employing Widrow and Hoff's LMS algorithm, is used to reduce the remainder of the interference, yielding an improvement in SNR. Clear ECGs have been obtained even with electrocautery equipment in operation, though the filtering process increases the complexity of the system.

Almenar et al. [15] implemented a single-input adaptive filter which requires a single input channel and is a combination of an adaptive impulse-correlated filter and a time-sequenced adaptive filter. This filter does not perform inter-beat averaging, but uses a normalised LMS (NLMS) algorithm to update the filter weights. The authors successfully applied the method to real ECG signals during stress tests and stated that their techniques could be applied to other fields involving signals with recurring statistics, such as radar and ultrasound non-destructive evaluation.

Christopher et al. [16] introduced Fourier analysis of biological signals to track the changes in evoked potentials (EP). They preferred this method because of the periodic and band-limited nature of the bio signals. The evoked response is modelled as a dynamic Fourier series and the Fourier coefficients are estimated adaptively by the least mean square algorithm. Approximate expressions have been developed for the estimation error and time constant of adaptation. A procedure for optimising the estimator performance is also presented. The effectiveness of the estimator in dealing with simulated, as well as actual, evoked responses is demonstrated. The Fourier coefficients are constant when EP is invariant, so LMS adaptation was used to vary the coefficients.

Allan et al. [17] analysed the mean square error of a Fourier linear combiner-based filter and showed that as the input SNR decreases, the MSE behaves better. An approach to prediction of respiration motion signals using LMS is given in [18]. In this paper, an improved version of normalised LMS and LMS algorithms using a Fast Lane Approach, based on parallel evaluation of several competing predictors, is presented. They were applied to respiratory motion data from motion-compensated radio surgery.

Adaptive electromyogram enhancement is presented in [19], and this recognises the applications of adaptive filtering in various biological signal enhancements. Applications of adaptive filtering include reducing the effects of respiration [21] and cancelling PLI and baseline wander [23, 25]. Cardiopulmonary resuscitation (CPR) artefacts caused by chest compressions and ventilations interfere with the rhythm diagnosis of automated external defibrillators, and CPR artefact removal by adaptive filtering is presented in [26]. A non-linear method is described by Ziaran et al. in [22], who developed an adaptive electromagnetic interference (EMI) filter for removing PLI. The dynamics of the algorithm make this act as a notch filter as it removes one frequency component. The authors claimed the filter as adaptive as it accommodates variations of characteristics in the desired output over time.

In one study [27], however, a steady-state convergence analysis for the LMS algorithm with deterministic reference inputs showed that the steady-state weight vector is biased, so the adaptive estimate does not approach the Wiener solution. To handle this drawback, another strategy, the block LMS (BLMS) algorithm [28], was considered for estimating the coefficients of the linear expansion. Here, the coefficient vector is updated only once every occurrence, based on a block gradient estimation. The BLMS algorithm has been proposed in the case of random reference inputs, when the input is stationary, the same steady state misadjustment and convergence speed as the LMS algorithm.

Poornachandra et al. [29] described a method for denoising and compression based on a sub-band adaptive technique. They tested it with normal and abnormal ECG signals; they added standard Gaussian noise, but no other artefacts were considered. Barros et al. [33] used an LMS algorithm to remove respiration noises and motion artefacts in Impedance Cardiography (ICG), a tool for assessing cardiac status.

In 2011, Rik Vullings et al. [4] proposed a sequential averaging filter that, in essence, adaptively varies the number of complexes included in the averaging, based on the characteristics of the ECG signal. It has the form of an adaptive Kalman filter. Jianbo Gao et al. [141] proposed an adaptive de-noising algorithm. Using chaotic Lorenz data and calculating root-mean-square-error, Lyapunov exponent, and correlation dimension, they proved that the adaptive algorithm more effectively reduces noise in the chaotic Lorenz system than does wavelet denoising with three different thresholding choices.

In the cardiology domain, ECG recording remains the most important, independent, objective, and non-invasive source of information for clinical evaluation of patients with chest pain and/or heart rhythm abnormalities [48]. The ability to monitor the cardiac activity of a distant patient ushers in a new era of wireless cardiology and telecardiology. As work in this field has intensified, many ambulatory devices have been reported recently. Boyle et al. [65] used a single lead ECG to measure respiration rate in an ambulatory environment. Dynamic monitoring of heart has become essential, and lightweight, wearable ECG recorders (W-ECGs) are recognised as more convenient than the standard Holter monitor, which restricts free movement. In [36] the authors developed a single lead W-ECG. It can store up to 48 hours' worth of signals, which can be downloaded to a personal computer via a serial port. In this paper, the authors characterised motion artefacts induced by body movement.

The typical telecardiology application described in [66] passes its signals from the remote patient to the hospital through different wireless protocols like SMS, MMS, HTTP and other custom socket routines. A patient with multiple conditions needs a special biotelemetry platform that can collect multiple health parameters and send them promptly to a remote health centre for diagnosis. To reduce mobile health costs, all such sensors should be very small, with low memory capacity but long battery duration. This type of bio-monitoring sensor network is implemented and presented in [67]. The main aspects reported in this paper are network embedded system design, network congestion reduction and network loss compensation. Various architectures and wireless sensor network-based estimation for biomedical signals are illustrated in [69, 70, 75].

Alesanco et al. [71] presented an absolute study of the use of wireless links for real-time telecardiac monitoring, considering both technical and clinical aspects, in order to provide recommendations for real-time monitoring that considered both channel parameters and the tolerance of cardiologists to the effects of interruptions introduced during transmission. By using extensive simulated wireless scenarios, the compressed ECG signal is monitored on reception.

But in these papers, less efforts have been made to reduce the computational complexity of the adaptive filter at the receiving end without affecting the signal quality. In this work, we propose various low complexity adaptive noise cancellers (ANCs) to filter different artefacts in ECG signals. For this, the input and the desired response signals are chosen in such a way that the filter output is the best least squared estimate of the ECG signal.

2.7. Conclusion

In this chapter, the basic principles of the adaptive filter and its properties, convergence rate, misadjustment, tracking and computational requirements are reviewed from literature and the necessary modifications to the adaptive noise canceller made according to the requirements for

ECG enhancement. The familiar LMS algorithm is discussed fully, as we used it as a reference algorithm for comparison with our proposed implementations. A basic adaptive filter structure for noise cancellation in ECG signals is introduced. The most important feature of adaptive filtering in biomedical signal processing is that it allows estimation of the underlying signal in the absence of a prior knowledge of the statistical nature of the signal or noise. Using this frame work, we develop different filter structures to remove diverse forms of noises like power line interference, baseline wander, muscle artefacts and electrode motion artefacts.

Chapter 3

Sign LMS Based Adaptive Filtering Techniques for the Removal of Noise in the ECG Signals

3.1. Introduction

In biomedical signal analysis when the input signal and artefacts are both stationary and their statistical characteristics are approximately known, an optimal filter like a Wiener filter or a matched filter can be used. In practical cases like biomedical signal analysis, a priori information is not available or when the signal or noise is non-stationary such an optimal design is not possible [12, 20]. In such a case adaptive filter has an ability to adjust their weight coefficients based on the incoming signal. Adaptation occurs through the modification of the parameters of the filter based on information of the incoming signal so that a given performance index is optimized. Thus, they require little or no prior knowledge of the signal or noise characteristics. Since no or almost no prior information is available, an adaptive filter requires an initial period for learning or adaptation. During this period, its performance is unsatisfactory. After initial adaptation the filter is supposed to act optimally while tracking the non-stationary changes in signal and artefacts [163].

Table 3.1. Summary of algorithms used in Chapter 3

S. No	Acronym	Name	Advantage
1.	LLMS	Leaky least mean square	Weight drift problem can be avoided and stability increases
2.	DZLMS	Dead zone least mean square	Diminish the problem of round off error
3.	LMF	Least mean fourth	Lower steady state error than LMS
4.	MLMS	Median least mean square	Smoothes the impulsive noise
5.	SR-LMS	Sign regressor least mean square	Single multiplication required and data is clipped
6.	S-LMS	Sign error least mean square	Error is clipped
7.	SS-LMS	Sign sign least mean square	Zero multiplications and both data, error is clipped
8.	SR-LLMS	Sign regressor leaky least mean square	Single multiplication required and data is clipped, Weight drift problem can be avoided and stability increases
9.	S-LLMS	Sign error leaky least mean square	Error is clipped, Weight drift problem can be avoided and stability increases
10.	SS-LLMS	Sign sign leaky least mean square	Zero multiplications and both data, error is clipped, Weight drift problem can be avoided and stability increases
11.	SR-DZLMS	Sign regressor dead zone least mean square	Single multiplication required and data is clipped, Diminish the problem of round off error
12.	S-DZLMS	Sign error dead zone least mean square	Error is clipped, Diminish the problem of round off error
13.	SS-DZLMS	Sign sign dead zone least mean square	Zero multiplications and both data, error is clipped, Diminish the problem of round off error
14.	SR-LMF	Sign regressor least mean fourth	Single multiplication required and data is clipped, Lower steady state error than LMS
15.	S-LMF	Sign error least mean fourth	Error is clipped, Lower steady state error than LMS
16.	SS-LMF	Sign sign least mean fourth	Zero multiplications and both data, error is clipped, Lower steady state error than LMS
17.	SR-MLMS	Sign regressor median least mean square	Single multiplication required and data is clipped, Smoothens the impulsive noise
18.	S-MLMS	Sign error median least mean square	Error is clipped, Smoothens the impulsive noise
19.	SS-MLMS	Sign sign median least mean square	Zero multiplications and both data, error are clipped, Smoothens the impulsive noise

(LMF) and Median LMS (MLMS). The efficiency of these algorithms for the removal of noise from ECG signals is given in results and discussions section.

LMS based adaptive algorithms make use of the factor that the error performance surface is a function of the filter weight vector. Thus, for each tap weight vector there exists a single value of the objective function which determines the state of the adaptive process. The idea is to iteratively update the tap weights in such a way that every new instance lies in the direction of the gradient. In this chapter we develop LMS based methods, in which the weight update equation is varied with respect to that of LMS. The fundamentals of these methods are taken from literature [76-80, 86, 96, 100, 158-160]. The summary of algorithms used in this chapter is given in Table 3.1.

We are investigating the performance of these methods under unconventional conditions, such as ECG signal with artefacts input, abrupt change of parameters or high level of noise. The aim of this Chapter is to provide an extensive comparison of methods. Here we consider five algorithms which can be straightly derived from the LMS algorithm namely, Leaky LMS (LLMS), Dead-Zone LMS (DZLMS), Least mean fourth.

3.2. Leaky LMS Algorithm

The LMS algorithm is used widely in numerous applications because of its simplicity. The direct implementation of LMS algorithm is sensitive to round-off errors and causes some other disturbances as the weight update equation is essentially an integrator. For example, inadequate excitation in the input sequence can result an unbounded parameter estimates. Since it is possible for these un-damped modes to become unstable, it is necessary for the stability of the LMS algorithm to force these modes to zero. By introducing a small leakage factor γ to the tap-weight vector should protect the algorithm from such numerical problems. The effect of introducing the leakage factor γ to force any un damped modes to become zero or force the tap weights to zero if either $e(n)$ or $\boldsymbol{x(n)}$ is zero [77]. This algorithm is known as the leaky LMS algorithm, and the parameter γ is referred to as the leak.

In ECG signal processing under critical conditions some of the samples in the ECG signal becomes zero, i.e., the excitation is inadequate. At these samples the weights vary drastically. The fluctuations in weights is called weight drift problem. By introducing a small leakage factor, we can overcome this problem. So here we make use of leaky LMS algorithm. The name stems from the fact that, when the input is turned off, the weight vector of the regular LMS algorithm stalls. With leaky LMS in the same scenario, the weight vector instead leaks out. It has been shown that leaky LMS can be used to improve stability in a finite-precision implementation, ameliorate the effects of non-persistent excitation, and reduce undesirable effects like stalling, bursting, etc. Detailed analysis of the performance of this algorithm is given in [76].

Now the weight update equation becomes,

$$\boldsymbol{w}(n+1) = (1-\mu\gamma)\boldsymbol{w}(n) + \mu e(n)\boldsymbol{x}(n) \tag{3.1}$$

In the above recursion it is chosen such that the product $\mu\gamma$ is greater than but close to 0. The leaky LMS algorithm (LLMS) has been used to improve the characteristics of an adaptive filter; which we exploit to efficiently cancel the noise from ECG signals, few are listed below [109].

1. Ill conditioned input signal i.e., it is useful for improving the convergence properties when the input correlation matrix is ill-conditioned. As a result, the input correlation matrix will exhibit unbalanced values on the main diagonal. In this manner we can increase the energy of values at the main diagonal and therefore regularize the correlation matrix.
2. Algorithm stalling when the correction term is too small.
3. Over flow due to finite-precision arithmetic.

3.3. Dead Zone LMS Algorithm

Small values of the error signal *e*(*n*) may represent disturbances or noise but may also result from numerical instability. In an ECG noise canceller these small errors and large errors causes additional filtering operations, lead to delay for making decision. In critical conditions the decision has to be make instantaneously. To avoid these additional computations, we need to set a threshold to error value. In signal processing applications the Dead Zone LMS (DZ-LMS) is used to diminish the problems of round-off errors. The algorithm applies dead zone nonlinearity and stops uploading the tap-weight vector when the error signal falls below some pre-defined threshold [158-160]. We use this property of DZ-LMS in filtering the ECG signal. This nonlinearity is defined as

$$g\{x\} = \begin{Bmatrix} x - d, x > d > 0 \\ 0, -d < x < d \\ x + d, x < -d \end{Bmatrix} \tag{3.2}$$

where *d* is threshold.

When applied to the error signal, it converts the LMS update recursion equation to

$$\boldsymbol{w}(n + 1) = \boldsymbol{w}(n) + \mu g\{e(n)\}\boldsymbol{x}(n) \tag{3.3}$$

3.4. Least Mean Fourth Algorithm

Adaptive filters based on higher order statistics are known to perform better than the mean square estimation employed in the Least-Mean Square algorithm in particular scenarios. In order to examine this, we developed different ANCs to remove PLI, BW, MA and EM from ECG signals. An algorithm based on the minimization of the fourth moment of the output estimation error, namely the Least-Mean Fourth (LMF) algorithm [108] is one such example. This algorithm is closely related to LMS algorithm. LMF algorithm tries to a higher power of the error signal, specifically the fourth order. The weight recursion for the LMF algorithm is shown as,

$$\boldsymbol{w}(n+1) = \boldsymbol{w}(n) + \mu e^3(n)\boldsymbol{x}(n) \tag{3.4}$$

LMF algorithm exhibits lower steady state error than the conventional LMS algorithm. This is due to the fact that the excess mean-square error of the LMS algorithm is dependent only on the second order moment of the noise. The second order moment, or variance of the noise evaluates to be the same for all the noise environments. In contrast, the excess mean-square error of the LMF algorithm depends on higher order moments of the noise that results in lower steady-state error as compared to the LMS algorithm. Recognizing this feature of the LMF algorithm, it was also known that the convergence behavior of the LMS and LMF algorithms is susceptible to the condition number, i.e., on the ratio of the maximum to the minimum eigen values of the input signal autocorrelation matrix.

To overcome this consequence of the ratio, the data normalization can be used, where the LMF recursion was modified to include an inverse norm of the input regressor. This gives in a fast convergence rate and good stability. However, this higher-order statistics of the error in the LMF algorithm requires smaller step-size to ensure stable adaptation [78]-[79].

3.5. Median LMS Algorithm

The performance of the LMS algorithm and its derivatives significantly degrades when subjected to input signals that are corrupted by impulsive noise, sometimes this leads to instability. In ECG signal processing this case occurs when the amplitude of the P wave increases due to abnormal heart rhythm. Smoothing the noisy gradient components using a nonlinear filter is a best remedy for this problem. This modification leads to median LMS. Computing the median of window size L + 1, for each component of the gradient vector, will smooth out the effect of impulsive noise [80]. If the input or reference signals are not corrupted with impulsive noise the performance of median LMS is same as that of conventional LMS, thus the extra computation cost of median LMS is not worth.

The weight update recursion is given by,

$$\boldsymbol{w}(n+1) = \boldsymbol{w}(n) + \mu . med_L[e(n)\boldsymbol{x}(n), e(n-1)\boldsymbol{x}(n-1) \ldots \ldots e(n-L)\boldsymbol{x}(n-L)] \tag{3.5}$$

The median function is interesting since it tends to reject single occurrence of large spikes of noise. These spikes would otherwise affect the estimates of w(n) and introduce impulsive errors. This property can be effectively utilized in situations, in which ECG signal is corrupted with PLI, BW, MA and EM like noises.

3.6. Extension To Sign Based Realizations of LMS Based Adaptive Filters

New algorithms that makes use of the signum (polarity) of either the error, the input signal, or both, have been derived from the various LMS based algorithms discussed above for the simplicity of implementation, enabling a significant reduction in computing time, particularly the time required for "multiply and accumulate" (MAC) operations [86]. Sign based treatment results in the reduction of computational complexity of the filter and hence suitable for biotelemetry applications. In this section we apply signum function to various algorithms and evaluate the performance in artefact removal from ECG signals. The sign-based algorithms enjoy the advantages of their LMS based versions, mentioned in the previous sections and reduced computational complexity due to signum function present in the algorithm. The performance of an adaptive filter mainly depends on the algorithm used for weight updating, Convergence analysis for LMS and Signed algorithms leads to a conclusion that, LMS algorithms are exponentially convergent, whereas the signed algorithms is linearly convergent. This makes convergence of the signed algorithms is slowest when the initial weight setting is far from the optimum [87, 90].

3.6.1. Sign Based LMS Algorithm

The derivation of these algorithms is similar to LMS algorithm up to (2.17). At this stage the recursion is modified by applying signum function. The most important members of this class of algorithms are: Signed Regressor Algorithm (SRA), Sign Algorithm (SA) and Sign-Sign Algorithm (SSA).

3.6.1.1. Sign-Regressor LMS Algorithm

The signed-regressor algorithm is obtained from the conventional LMS recursion by replacing the tap-input vector **x**(n) with the vector Sign{**x**(n)}, where the sign function is applied to the vector **x**(n) on an element-by-element basis. This is also called as clipped LMS as we are clipping the input data. The signed-regressor recursion is then

$$\boldsymbol{w}(n+1) = \boldsymbol{w}(n) + \mu e(n) Sign\{\boldsymbol{x}(n)\} \tag{3.6}$$

where

$$Sign\{\boldsymbol{x}(n)\} = \begin{Bmatrix} 1: \boldsymbol{x}(n) > 0 \\ 0: \boldsymbol{x}(n) = 0 \\ -1: \boldsymbol{x}(n) < 0 \end{Bmatrix} \tag{3.7}$$

The *k*th coefficient in the sign of the data vector may be written as follows:

$$Sign\{\boldsymbol{x}(n-k)\} = \frac{x(n-k)}{|x(n-k)|} \tag{3.8}$$

In the normalized LMS algorithm where the weight vector is normalized by $||\mathbf{x}(n)||^2$, the sign regressor algorithm individually normalized each coefficient of the weight vector so this performs better than the other algorithms.

3.6.1.2. Sign Error LMS Algorithm

This algorithm is obtained from the conventional LMS recursion by replacing *e(n)* with its sign. This is also called as pilot LMS. This leads to the following recursion:

$$\boldsymbol{w}(n+1) = \boldsymbol{w}(n) + \mu Sign\{e(n)\}\boldsymbol{x}(n) \tag{3.9}$$

Because of the replacement of *e(n)*, implementation of the recursion become cheaper than the conventional LMS recursion, especially in high speed application where a hardware implementation of the adaptation recursion may be necessary. The simplification in the sign-error algorithm comes when the step size chosen to be a power of two, $\mu = 2^{-l}$, so that no multiplication would be required for implementing the recursion. A set of shift and add/subtract operation would suffice to update the filter tap weights.

3.6.1.3. Sign-Sign LMS Algorithm

The sign-sign algorithm combines the sign and signed-regressor recursions resulting in the following recursion:

$$\boldsymbol{w}(n+1) = \boldsymbol{w}(n) + \mu Sign\{e(n)\}Sign\{\boldsymbol{x}(n)\} \tag{3.10}$$

This is also called as zero forcing LMS because of zero multiplications in the implementation.

The performance of the signed regressor algorithm is slightly worse than the conventional algorithm. However, the sign and sign-sign algorithms are both much slower than the conventional LMS algorithm. Their convergence behavior is also rather peculiar. They converge very slowly at the beginning, but speed up as the MSE level drops. This can be explained as follows.

Consider the sign algorithm recursion and it may be written as,

$$\mathbf{w}(n + 1) = \mathbf{w}(n) + \mu\{\mathbf{x}(n)\}\{e(n)/|e(n)|\} \quad (3.11)$$

Since $Sign[e(n)] = e(n)/|e(n)|$

This is rearranged as,

$$\mathbf{w}(n + 1) = \mathbf{w}(n) + [\frac{\mu}{|e(n)|}]\mathbf{x}(n)e(n) \quad (3.12)$$

The above equation reveals that the sign algorithm may be thought as an LMS algorithm with a variable step size parameter, $\mu'(n) = \{\mu/|e(n)|\}$. The step size parameter $\mu'(n)$ increases, on an average, as the sign algorithm converges, since $e(n)$ decreases in magnitude. Thus, to keep the sign algorithm stable, with a small steady state error, a very small step size has to be used. A small μ leads to an equally small value for $\mu'(n)$ in the initial portion of the sign algorithm. As a result, the algorithm initially converges slowly. However, as the algorithm converges and $e(n)$ becomes smaller in magnitude, the step size $\mu'(n)$ becomes larger, leads to a faster convergence. Moreover, the sign present in the algorithm and setting μ to a value of power of two, the hardware implementation is highly simplified (shift and add / subtract operation only).

In the same manner the behavior of signed regressor algorithm can be analyzed. In this case each tap of the filter is controlled by a separate variable step size parameter. For example, the step size parameter of the ith tap of the filter at the nth iteration is$\mu_i'(n) = \{\mu/|x(n-i)|\}$, where μ is a common parameter to all taps. The fundamental difference between the variable step parameter $\mu_i'(n)$s here and that in sign algorithm is that in the present case the variations in the $\mu'(n)$ is independent of the filter convergence. Here the selection of step size is based on the average size of

$x(n)$. This leads to a more homogeneous convergence of the signed regressor algorithm when compared with sign algorithm.

3.6.2. Sign Based Leaky LMS Algorithm

This is an extension of Leaky LMS algorithm described in section 3.1. All the arguments made in section 3.6.1 are applicable to this case except the weight update equation differs. In this case we use the recursion given by (3.1). Now the three versions of sign-based algorithms are written as follows.

The sign regressor Leaky LMS (SRLLMS), in this case we apply signum function to data. According to (3.7) after applying this function data becomes -1 or 0 or 1. This can be written as,

$$\mathbf{w}(n + 1) = (1 - \mu\gamma)\mathbf{w}(n) + \mu e(n)Sign\{\mathbf{x}(n)\} \tag{3.13}$$

Because of the signum function, as in (3.8) data normalization takes place. So this algorithm enjoys the advantages good stability and better filtering, convergence.

Similarly application of the signum function to error term in (3.1) that yields sign Leaky LMS (SLLMS) and is given by,

$$\mathbf{w}(n + 1) = (1 - \mu\gamma)\mathbf{w}(n) + \mu Sign\{e(n)\}\mathbf{x}(n) \tag{3.14}$$

If we apply signum for both data and error part of (3.1) that results sign sign Leaky LMS (SSLLMS) given by,

$$\mathbf{w}(n + 1) = (1 - \mu\gamma)\mathbf{w}(n) + \mu Sign\{e(n)\}Sign\{\mathbf{x}(n)\} \tag{3.15}$$

Here because of the signum function for both data and error, some residual noise remains in the filtering process. At the same time computational complexity greatly reduced as a result of (3.7). Among the three, SRLLMS performs better because of the leakage term and data normalization involved because of the signum function. Moreover, its computational complexity is also reduced by using signum function.

3.6.3. Sign Based Dead Zone LMS Algorithm

DZLMS is one of the common modifications to adaptive algorithms, incorporates the error non-linearity. Because of this the function 'g' in (3.2) is insensitive to small errors, which are sometimes presumed due to noise. Actually, in DZLMS under goes error round off due to the function 'g'. The three versions of simplified algorithms SRA, SA, SSA in combination with DZLMS results sign regressor DZLMS (SRDZLMS), signed DZLMS (SDZLMS) and sign sign DZLMS (SSDZLMS) respectively. These results due to the combination of (3.3) and (3.6), (3.9) and (3.10) and yields as follows.

The SRDZLMS is given by,

$$\boldsymbol{w}(n+1) = \boldsymbol{w}(n) + \mu g\{e(n)\} Sign\{\boldsymbol{x}(n)\} \tag{3.16}$$

Similarly, SDZLMS and SSDZLMS are given by,

$$\boldsymbol{w}(n+1) = \boldsymbol{w}(n) + \mu Sign\{g[e(n)]\}\boldsymbol{x}(n) \tag{3.17}$$

$$\boldsymbol{w}(n+1) = \boldsymbol{w}(n) + \mu Sign\{g[e(n)]\}Sign\{\boldsymbol{x}(n)\} \tag{3.18}$$

In these two algorithms (3.2) is rounded to -1 or 0 or 1.

3.6.4. Sign Based Least Mean Fourth Algorithm

LMF algorithm is a basic version of higher order adaptive filter. The combination of LMF (3.4) with SRA, SA and SSA gives SRLMF, SLMF and SSLMF respectively. These are given as follows.

$$\boldsymbol{w}(n+1)=\boldsymbol{w}(n)+\mu e^{3}(n)Sign\{\boldsymbol{x}(n)\} \tag{3.19}$$

$$\boldsymbol{w}(n+1)=\boldsymbol{w}(n)+\mu Sign\{e^{3}(n)\}\boldsymbol{x}(n) \tag{3.20}$$

$$\boldsymbol{w}(n+1)=\boldsymbol{w}(n)+\mu Sign\{e^{3}(n)\}Sign\{\boldsymbol{x}(n)\} \tag{3.21}$$

From (3.19) and (3.20) it is noted that SLMF and SSLMF are same as SLMS and SSLMS.

3.6.5. Sign Based Median LMS Algorithm

The median filter is suitable if input signal is contaminated with a sudden impulsive noise. From (3.5) it is clear that the computational complexity is higher than the conventional LMS algorithm. Applying signum function to (3.5) significantly reduces computation cost. Here we apply signum function with three combinations mentioned in SRA, SA and SSA. These result SRMLMS, SMLMS and SSMLMS algorithms.

The SRMLMS is given by,

$$\boldsymbol{w}(n+1)=\boldsymbol{w}(n)+\mu.med_{L}[e(n)Sign\{\boldsymbol{x}(n)\},e(n-1)Sign\{\boldsymbol{x}(n-1)\}\ldots e(n-L)Sign\{\boldsymbol{x}(n-L)\}] \tag{3.22}$$

The SMLMS is given by,

$$\boldsymbol{w}(n+1)=\boldsymbol{w}(n)+\mu.med_{L}[Sign\{e(n)\}\boldsymbol{x}(n),Sign\{e(n-1)\}\boldsymbol{x}(n-1)\ldots Sign\{e(n-L)\}\boldsymbol{x}(n-L)] \tag{3.23}$$

The SSMLMS is given by,

$$\boldsymbol{w}(n+1)=\boldsymbol{w}(n)+\mu.med_{L}[Sign\{e(n)\}Sign\{\boldsymbol{x}(n)\},Sign\{e(n-1)\}Sign\{\boldsymbol{x}(n-1)\}\ldots Sign\{e(n-L)\}Sign\{\boldsymbol{x}(n-L)\}] \tag{3.24}$$

3.7. Computational Complexity Issues

Generally, to estimate and compare algorithm complexity number of multiplications required to complete the operation is taken as a measure. However, most of the DSP's have a built-in hardware support for multiplication and accumulation (MAC) operations. Usually they perform this operation in a single instruction cycle as well as addition or subtraction. In this work we are not trying to provide a precise analysis of a computational complexity, rather we concentrate on presenting a comparison between different adaptive algorithms. The computational complexity figures required to compute all the LMS based adaptive filters and their sign-based realizations are summarized in Table 3.2, offers significant reduction in the number of operations required for LMS algorithm. Further, as these sign-based algorithms are largely free from multiplication operation, these algorithms provide elegant means for removing the noise from the ECG signals. For example, LMS algorithm L + 1 multiplications and L + 1 addition are required to compute the weight update equation (2.17), where L is the length of the filter. In case of signed regressor algorithm only one multiplication is required to compute $\mu e(n)$. Whereas other two signed LMS algorithms does not require multiplication if we choose μ value a power of 2. In these cases, multiplication becomes shift operation which is less complex in practical realizations. In SSA we apply signum to both data and vector, and then we add μ to weight vector with addition with sign check (ASC) operation.

Table 3.2. Computational complexity of various LMS based algorithms

S. No.	Algorithm	Multiplications	Additions
1.	LMS	L + 1	L + 1
2.	LLMS	2L + 2	L + 1
3.	DZLMS	L + 1	L + 1
4.	LMF	L + 3	L + 1
5.	MLMS	L + 1	L + 1

Table 3.3. Computational complexity of sign-based variants of LMS algorithms

S. No.	Algorithm	Multiplications	Additions	ASC
1.	SR-LMS	1	L + 1	NIL
2.	S-LMS	L	L + 1	NIL
3.	SS-LMS	NIL	NIL	L + 1
4.	SR-LLMS	L + 2	L + 1	NIL
5.	S-LLMS	L	L + 1	NIL
6.	SS-LLMS	NIL	NIL	L + 1
7.	SR-DZLMS	1	L + 1	NIL
8.	S-DZLMS	L	L + 1	NIL
9.	SS-DZLMS	NIL	NIL	L + 1
10.	SR-LMF	3	L + 1	NIL
11.	S-LMF	L	L + 1	NIL
12.	SS-LMF	NIL	NIL	L + 1
13.	SR-MLMS	1	L + 1	NIL
14.	S-MLMS	L	L + 1	NIL
15.	SS-MLMS	NIL	NIL	L + 1

From Table 3.3 it is clear that all the sign regressor algorithms has a smaller number of multiplications, because of the sign term applied to data vector, i.e., all the elements of the data vector become -1 or 0 or 1, so that multiplications are greatly reduced. In the case of sign applied to error, there is no significant change in number of multiplications, where as in sign-sign algorithm signum function is applied to both data vector and error term, therefore no multiplication is needed to compute the weight update equation, all the computations can be carried with addition operations with sign check.

3.8. Convergence Analysis

The convergence curves for various LMS variant adaptive algorithms discussed in the previous sections are shown in Figure 3.1. These curves are plotted between MSE and number of iterations. MSE is calculated using (2.1), i.e., $\xi = E\{|e(n)|^2\}$. This simulation is done using

MATLAB. In this code we, MSE is calculated for each sample for 4000 iterations and the average value is taken for the characterization. These curves are obtained during the adaptive power line interference cancellation using various ANCs individually with a adaptive filter of length 5, random variance of 0.01 and step size 0.01. From Figure 3.1 it is clear that, among all the algorithms LLMS outperforms. The performance of MLMS, DLMS, and LMF are comparable to each other and superior to LMS. The Figure 3.2 to Figure 3.6 shows the convergence curves for sign LMS based algorithms. Due to the normalization factor in (3.8) the performance of the sign regressor version of LMS algorithms is slightly inferior to the corresponding non-signed version of the algorithm; the corresponding convergence curve is shown in Figure 3.2. The signed algorithms will always exhibit suboptimal convergence performance when compared to their conventional realizations since they tend to reject some information in exchange for lower complexity. The same phenomenon can be observed for all signed versions of LLMS, DZLMS, LMF and MLMS algorithms.

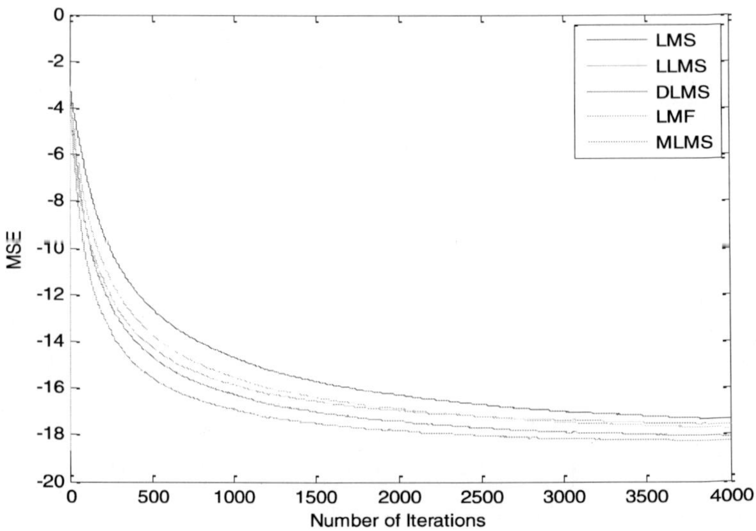

Figure 3.1. Convergence curves of LMS based algorithms.

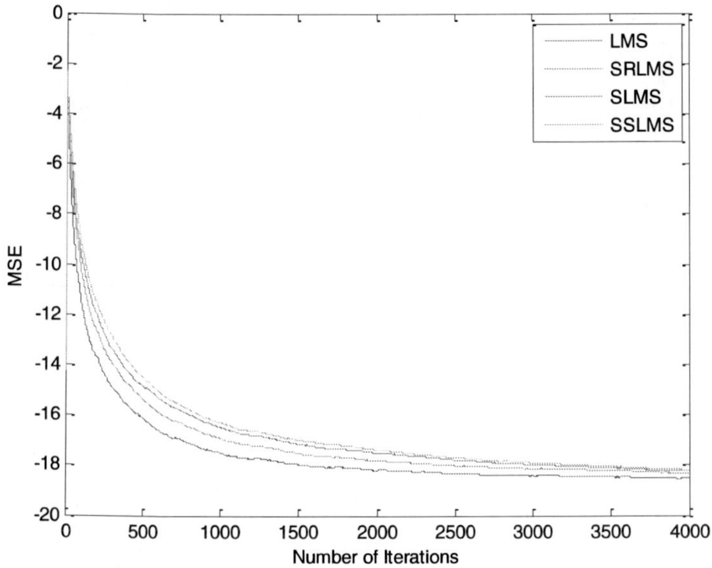

Figure 3.2. Convergence curves of sign based LMS algorithms.

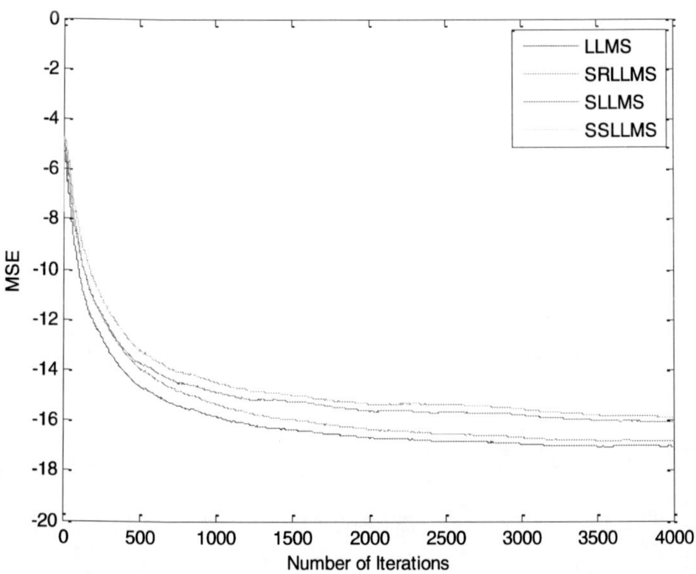

Figure 3.3. Convergence curves of sign based LLMS algorithms.

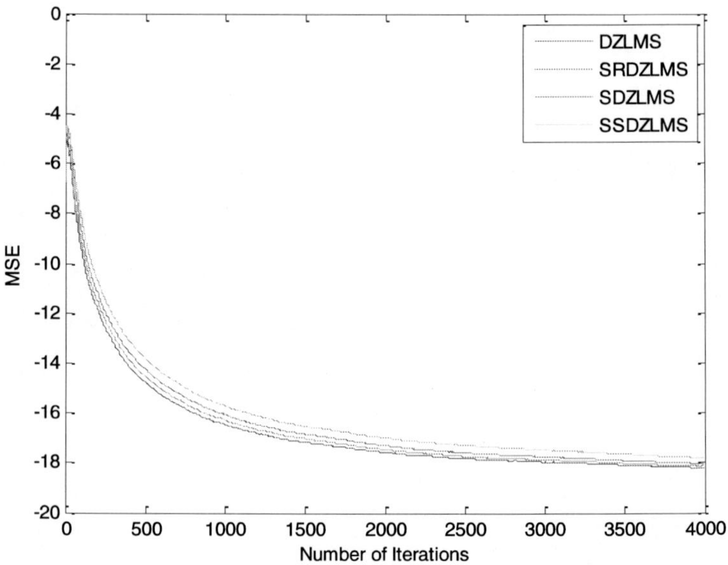

Figure 3.4. Convergence curves of sign based DZLMS algorithms.

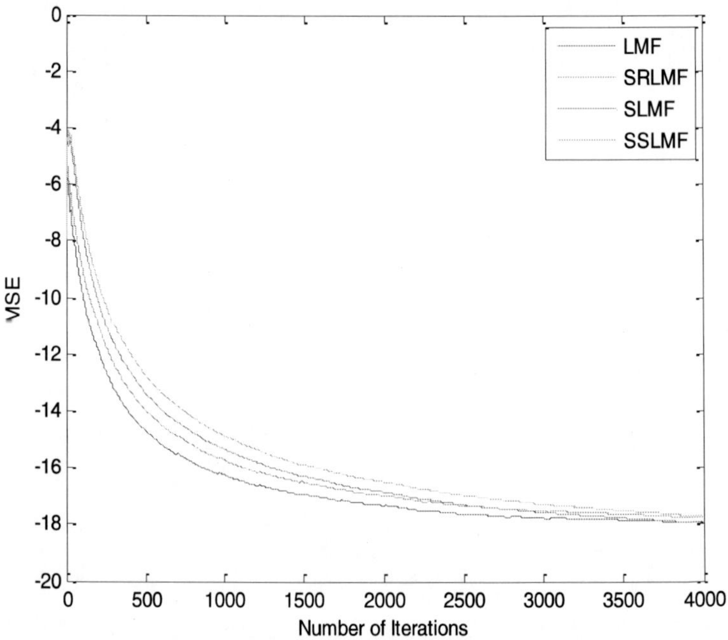

Figure 3.5. Convergence curves of sign based LMF algorithms.

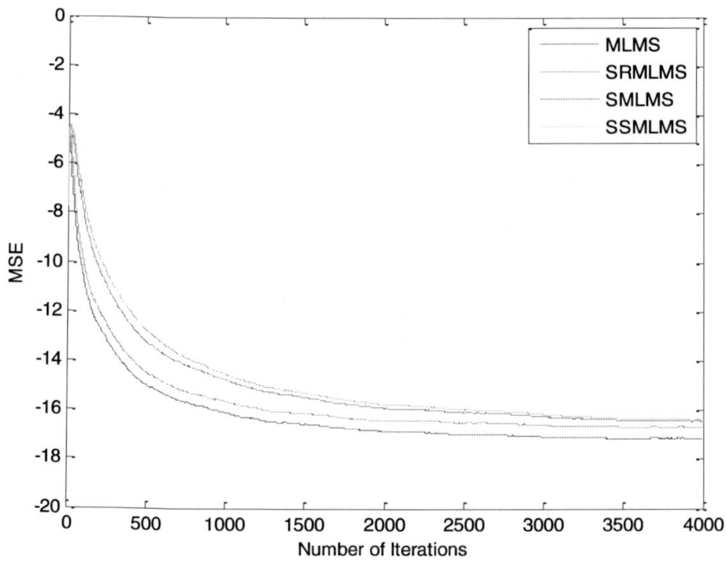

Figure 3.6. Convergence curves of sign based MLMS algorithms.

3.9. Results and Discussions

To test the ability of the various gradient based adaptive algorithms and their sign-based realizations discussed in this chapter we performed various experiments on real ECG signals with a wide variety of wave morphologies. We used the benchmark Massachusetts Institute of Technology and Boston's Beth Israel Hospital (MIT-BIH) arrhythmia database ECG [110] records for our work research.

The MIT-BIH Arrhythmia Database contains 48 half-hour excerpts of two-channel ambulatory ECG recordings, obtained from 47 subjects studied by the BIH Arrhythmia Laboratory ages 23 years to 89 years. Twenty-three recordings were chosen at random from a set of 4000 24-hour ambulatory ECG recordings collected from a mixed population of inpatients (about 60%) and outpatients (about 40%) at Boston's Beth Israel Hospital; the remaining 25 recordings were selected from the same set to include less common but clinically significant arrhythmias that would not be well-represented in a small random sample.

The recordings were digitized at 360 samples per second per channel with 11-bit resolution over a 10-mV range. About half (25 of 48 complete records, and reference annotation files for all 48 records) of this database has been freely available online since Physio Net's inception in September 1999. The 23 remaining signal files, which had been available on the MIT-BIH Arrhythmia Database online since February 2005.

The ECG recordings were made using Del Mar Avionics model 445 two-channel reel-to-reel Holter recorders, and the analog signals were recreated for digitization using a Del Mar Avionics model 660 playback unit. The computers used for digitization were designed and built in our laboratory, including the tape-drive controllers and the analog-to-digital converter (ADC) interfaces; they used then state-of-the-art 1 MHz 8-bit CPUs and 11-bit offset binary ADCs. The digitization rate (360 samples per second per channel) was chosen to accommodate the use of simple digital notch filters to remove 60 Hz (mains frequency) interference [161, [162].

In our experiments we have considered a dataset of five ECG records: data100, data105, data108, data203 and data228 to ensure the consistency of results, the simulation results for data 105 are shown in this work. In these experiments we have used first 4000 samples of the ECG signals. All the experiments were performed for 10 times and average values are tabulated. The length of the adaptive filter is chosen as 5, a random noise of variance 0.01 is added to the signals, which resembles the channel noise, the step size μ is taken as 0.01. For evaluating the performance of the proposed filter structures we have measured the signal-to-noise ratio improvement (SNRI) in decibels (dBs) using MATLAB program based on the (3.25) and compared with conventional LMS algorithm.

$$SNRI[db] = SNR_{output} - SNR_{input} = 10log\left(\frac{\sum_i |x_d(n) - x(n)|^2}{\sum_i |x_n(n) - x(n)|^2}\right) \quad (3.25)$$

where x denotes the clean ECG, x_d is the denoised signal and x_n represents the noisy ECG signal.

The signal powers are taken over the length of the signal, in this case that is 4000. Each experiment is performed for ten times and average value is taken, again the process is repeated for the five signals in the dataset considered and average value is taken. Similarly, the parameters MSE, M_{ad} and EMSE are measured using MATLAB programs based on the (2.1), (2.2) and (2.4) and average of ten times is tabulated for respective type of artefact.

For all the figures *number of samples* is taken on x-axis and *amplitude* on y-axis, unless stated. Various adaptive filter structures similar to shown in Figure 2.3 are implemented using LMS, LLMS, DZLMS, LMF, MLMS algorithms and their sign based (SRA, SA and SSA) versions. In our experiments, we have considered four dominant artefacts, namely Power Line Interference (PLI), Baseline Wander (BW), Muscle Artefacts (MA) and Electrode Motion artefacts (EM).

3.9.1. Noise Generator

The reference signal n_2 shown in Figure 2.3 is taken from noise generator. The noise generator first measures the input ECG signal power and produces the corresponding additive noise with a assigned signal to noise ratio (SNR). A synthetic PLI with 1mv amplitude is simulated for PLI cancellation. No harmonics are synthesized. In order to test the filtering capability in non-stationary environment we have considered real BW, MA and EM noises with a random noise of variance 0.01 to resemble the channel noise. The developed ANCs are tested with real noise obtained from MIT-BIH Normal Sinus Rhythm Database (NSRDB) and Noise Stress Test Database (NSTDB) [111, 112]. This database was recorded at a sampling rate of 128Hz from 18 subjects with no significant arrhythmias [161, 162]. A random noise with variance of 0.01 is generated, which resemble the channel noise. The input SNR for the above non-stationary noise is taken as 1.25dB. In the ANCs developed using sign-based algorithms because of the sign present in the recursion some tiny noise remains along the ST segment of the ECG signal. In order to extract the residual noise a tiny sinusoidal noise is added to the noise reference signal. This improves the performance of the filter. The same noise generator is used with the ANCs developed in the next chapters.

3.9.2. Adaptive Power-Line Interference Cancellation

This experiment demonstrates PLI cancellation, i.e., stationary noise cancellation. The input to the filter is ECG signal corrupted with a PLI of amplitude 1mv, frequency 60Hz and sampled at 200Hz. The reference signal is synthesized sinusoidal noise generated in the noise generator; the output of the filter is recovered signal. The developed MATLAB based ANCs have the same structure shown in Figure 2.3. The contaminated ECG signal is applied as input $x(n) = s_1 + n_1$, the correlated noise reference is applied as n_2 and the output is y(n). Five filter structures are implemented using LMS, LLMS, DLMS, LMF and MLMS algorithms. The simulation results are shown in Figure 3.7. In the simulated model initially, the weight vector is taken as a null vector. At the initial stage of the filtering the error is maximum, so that the adaptation is slow; this is clear from the convergence characteristics as well as from Figure 3.7, in which some noise component is present in the filtered signal. As number of feedback loops is going this error decreases because of the adaptation of the weight vector in accordance of the input noisy signal. The process will continue until the error value becomes minimum, i.e., the reference signal becomes closely correlated with the noise component in the ECG signal. Finally, the noise component is getting subtracted due to the trained reference signal because of the adaptive filter. The same analysis can be applied to all the adaptive noise cancellers. The performance of the various algorithms is measure in terms of SNRI by using the (3.1), averaged for ten times for each signal and tabulated in Table 3.4.

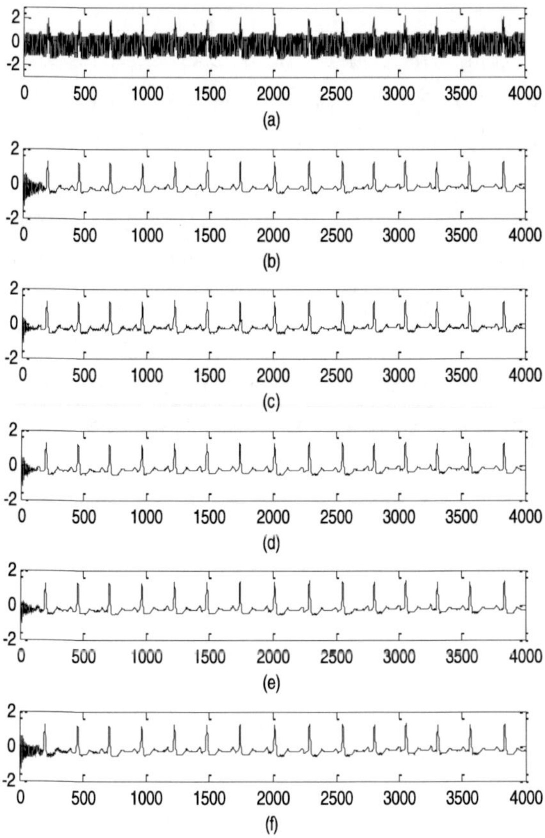

Figure 3.7. Typical filtering results for PLI cancellation using LMS based adaptive filtering techniques: (a) ECG signal with PLI, (b) recovered signal using LMS algorithm, (c) recovered signal using LLMS algorithm, (d) recovered signal using DZLMS algorithm, (e) recovered signal using LMF algorithm, (f) recovered signal using MLMS algorithm.

Table 3.4. SNRI contrast of LMS based adaptive algorithms for PLI removal

S. No	Record No	LMS	LLMS	DZLMS	LMF	MLMS
1.	100	7.7068	8.8039	8.1679	8.1225	8.42886
2.	105	7.7567	8.7544	8.0277	8.3485	8.1255
3.	108	7.7684	8.8393	8.3747	8.6694	8.0647
4.	203	7.7523	7.8763	7.4213	7.4479	8.4461
5.	228	7.0637	8.7811	8.1304	8.1723	8.3131
Average SNRI		7.6095	8.6110	8.0244	8.1521	8.2756

From Table 3.4 it is clear that LLMS algorithm achieves maximum SNRI with an average SNRI over the dataset is 8.6110 dBs, MLMS gets 8.2756 dBs, LMF gets 8.1521dBs and DZLMS gets 8.0244dBs, whereas the conventional LMS algorithm gets 7.6095 dBs. These values correlate with the convergence characteristics shown in Figure 3.1. The excess means square error (EMSE) and misadjustment (M_{ad}) due to various ANCs in different artefact environments are calculated using (2.4) and (2.2) are calculated and tabulated in Table 3.12. In evidence with SNRI and convergence characteristics among all the algorithms lower EMSE and M_{ad} is observed in LLMS based ANC, for the remaining algorithms the order of lower EMSE and M_{ad} is MLMS, LMF, DZLMS and LMS respectively.

Table 3.5. SNRI contrast of sign based adaptive algorithms for PLI removal

S.No.	Algorithm	Record No. 100	Record No. 105	Record No. 108	Record No. 203	Record No. 228	Average SNRI
1.	SRLMS	7.3809	7.2466	7.3738	7.3120	7.3840	7.3394
2.	SLMS	6.8429	6.7186	6.8391	7.2434	7.3828	7.0053
3.	SSLMS	6.0202	6.5759	6.3044	7.0479	7.3755	6.6647
4.	SRLLMS	8.2234	8.0252	8.2263	8.0181	8.2555	8.1497
5.	SLLMS	3.8340	5.4982	5.1533	6.5846	6.2435	5.4627
6.	SSLLMS	2.5796	4.5739	4.1763	5.5815	5.3270	4.4476
7.	SRDZLMS	7.6657	7.5452	7.7076	7.4673	7.7561	7.6283
8.	SDZLMS	7.3626	7.2636	7.2838	7.2086	7.474	7.3185
9.	SSDZLMS	6.2056	6.1016	6.3328	6.1579	6.0788	6.1753
10.	SRLMF	7.2983	7.4311	7.8886	7.6940	7.2870	7.5198
11.	SLMF	6.8429	6.7186	6.8391	7.2434	7.3828	7.0053
12.	SSLMF	6.0202	6.5759	6.3044	7.0479	7.3755	6.6647
13.	SRMLMS	7.3972	7.3527	7.3937	7.4761	7.6110	7.4461
14.	SMLMS	5.5058	6.6645	6.6926	6.9020	7.3983	6.6330
15.	SSMLMS	4.8423	6.1516	6.1415	6.4023	6.5438	6.0163

To enjoy the less computational complexity the LMS variant adaptive algorithms are combined with signed algorithms and results several algorithms. These are SRLMS, SLMS, SSLMS, SRLLMS, SLLMS, SSLLMS, SRDZLMS, SDZLMS, SSDZLMS, SRLMF, SLMF, SSLMF, SRMLMS, SMLMS and SSMLMS. Using these algorithms various ANCs are developed and tested for adaptive PLI removal. The filtering results are as follows from Figure 3.8 to Figure 3.12.

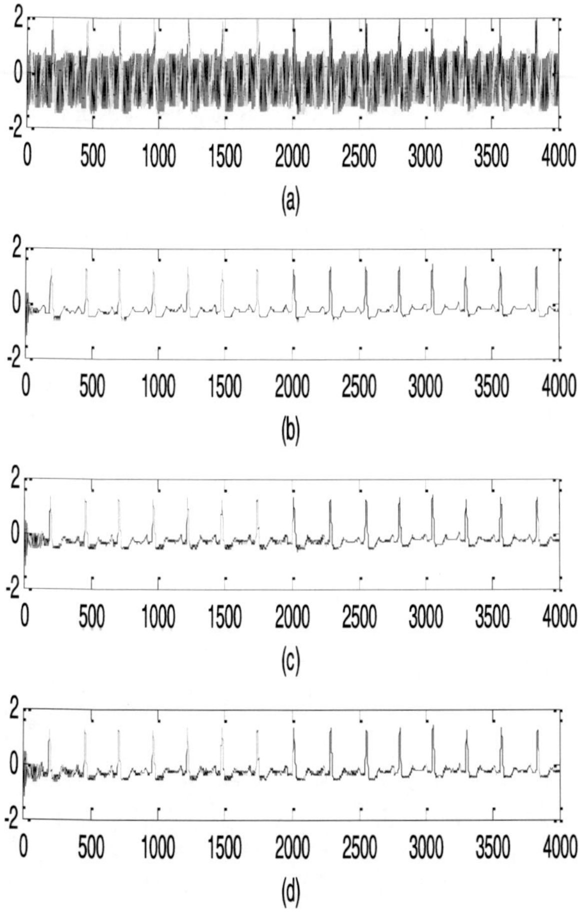

Figure 3.8. Typical filtering results for PLI cancellation using sign based LMS algorithm: (a) ECG signal with PLI, (b) recovered signal using SRLMS algorithm, (c) recovered signal using SLMS algorithm, (d) recovered signal using SSLMS algorithm.

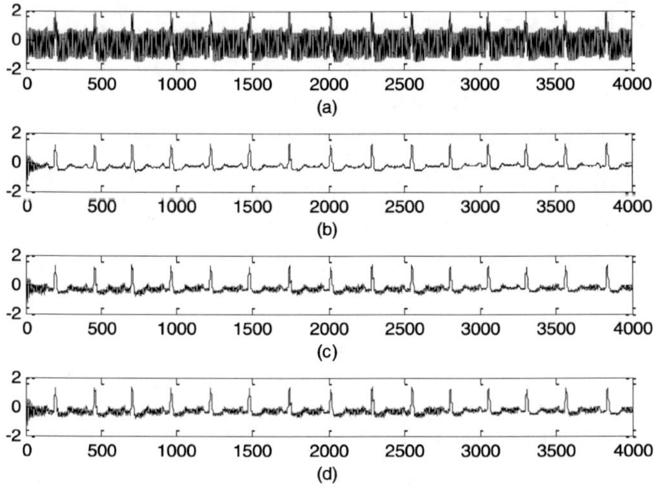

Figure 3.9. Typical filtering results for PLI cancellation using sign based LLMS algorithm: (a) ECG signal with PLI, (b) recovered signal using SRLLMS algorithm, (c) recovered signal using SLLMS algorithm, (d) recovered signal using SSLLMS algorithm.

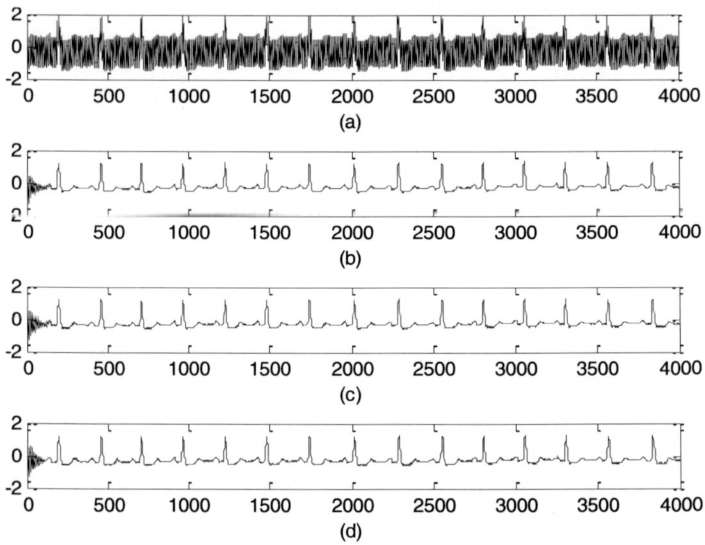

Figure 3.10. Typical filtering results for PLI cancellation using sign based DZLMS algorithm: (a) ECG signal with PLI, (b) recovered signal using SRDZLMS algorithm, (c) recovered signal using SDZLMS algorithm, (d) recovered signal using SSDZLMS algorithm.

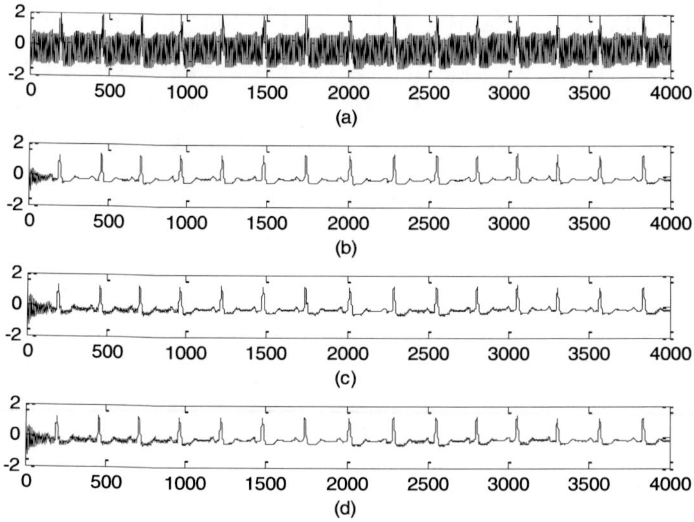

Figure 3.11. Typical filtering results for PLI cancellation using sign based LMF algorithm: (a) ECG signal with PLI, (b) recovered signal using SRLMF algorithm, (c) recovered signal using SLMF algorithm, (d) recovered signal using SSLMF algorithm.

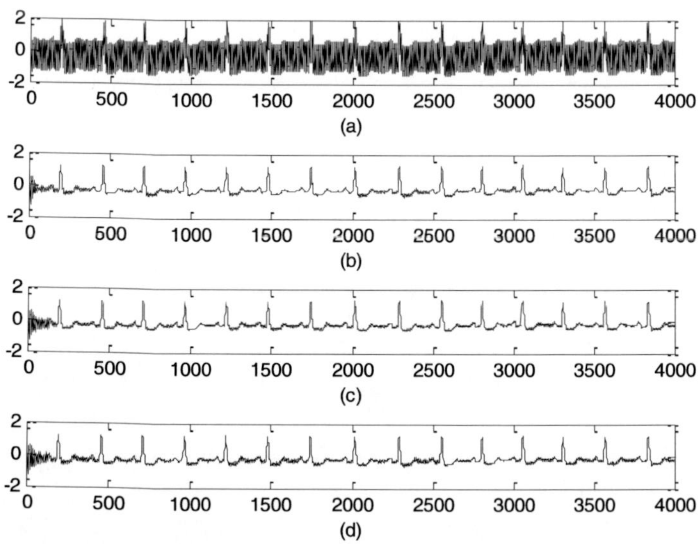

Figure 3.12. Typical filtering results for PLI cancellation using sign based MLMS algorithm: (a) ECG signal with PLI, (b) recovered signal using SRMLMS algorithm, (c) recovered signal using SMLMS algorithm, (d) recovered signal using SSMLMS algorithms.

The SNRI contrast of various sign-based algorithms for PLI removal is given in Table 3.5. Among all the algorithms SRMLMS gets first place with an average SNRI of 8.1497 dBs, the next place goes to SRDZLMS with a SNRI of 7.6283dBs. Whereas the conventional LMS algorithm gets 7.6095 dBs. Therefore, from the SNRI measurements it is clear that all sign regressor based algorithms achieves SNRI very close to that of LMS algorithm. Here it has to be noted that sign regressor based algorithms needs reduced number of multiplications by an amount equal to the filter length than its LMS based algorithm. The signed version of all algorithms gets SNRI less than their SRA but greater than SSA, here in the case of SA the number of multiplications required are approximately equal to the corresponding LMS based realization, whereas SSA requires no multiplications and it needs ASC operations only.

3.9.3. Adaptive Baseline Wander Removal

This experiment is developed for BW cancellation, which is a non-stationary noise cancellation. The input to the filter is ECG signal is contaminated with respiration baseline wander; this is applied to a noise canceller shown in Figure 2.3. The reference signal is a real BW obtained from MIT-BIH Noise Stress Test Database. Various filter structures are implemented using LMS, LLMS, DLMS, LMF and MLMS algorithms. These simulation results are shown in Figure 3.13.

The SNRI for various filtering methods is shown in Table 3.6. From SNR calculations it is clear that DZLMS effectively filters BW noise, it got an average SNRI of 3.9099 dBs, LMF gets 3.9080 dBs, LLMS gets 3.1006 dBs, MLMS get 3.0470 dBs whereas the conventional LMS gets 2.7488 dBs. The excess mean square error (EMSE) and misadjustment (M_{ad}) due to various ANCs in different artefact environments are measured using MATLAB programs written based on (2.4) and (2.2) and are tabulated in Table 3.12. To enjoy the less computational complexity the five LMS based adaptive algorithms are combined with signed algorithms and results fifteen algorithms. These are SR-LMS, S-LMS, SS-LMS, SR-LLMS, S-

LLMS, SS-LLMS, SR-DZLMS, S-DZLMS, SS-DZLMS, SR-LMF, S-LMF, SS-LMF, SR-MLMS, S-MLMS and SS-MLMS. Using these algorithms ANCs are developed and tested for removal of BW. The filtering results are as follows from Figure 3.14 to Figure 3.18.

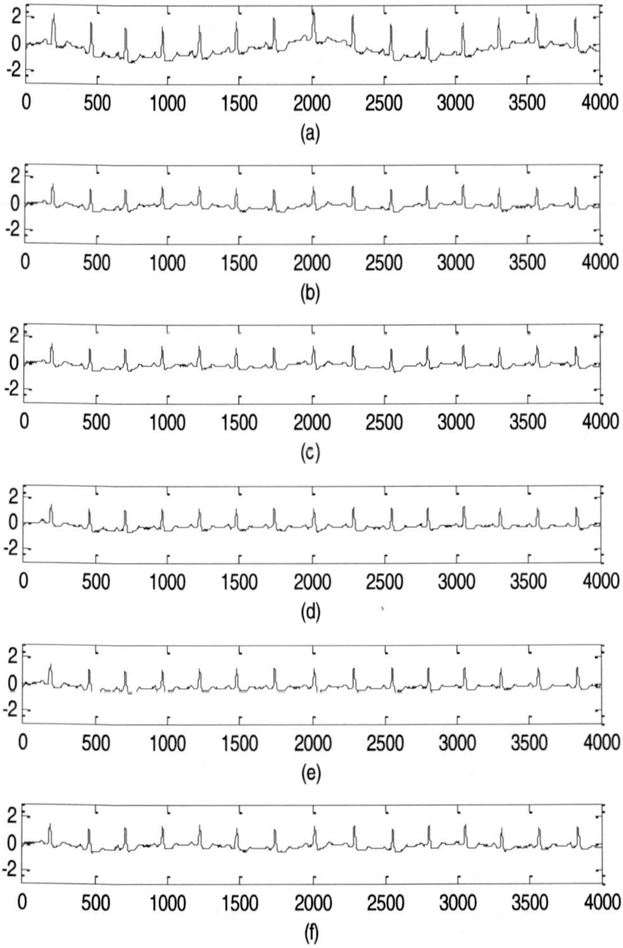

Figure 3.13. Typical filtering results for BW cancellation using LMS based adaptive filtering techniques: (a) ECG signal with real BW, (b) recovered signal using LMS algorithm, (c) recovered signal using LLMS algorithm, (d) recovered signal using DLMS algorithm, (e) recovered signal using LMF algorithm, (f) recovered signal using MLMS algorithm.

Table 3.6. SNRI contrast of adaptive algorithms for the removal of BW

S. No	Record No	LMS	LLMS	DZLMS	LMF	MLMS
1.	100	2.1986	2.2389	4.5031	4.4444	2.3247
2.	105	3.4080	3.9133	4.7512	4.9814	3.7849
3.	108	2.2791	2.8995	3.7164	3.6113	2.7808
4.	203	2.6438	2.9489	2.9522	3.2555	2.8411
5.	228	3.2148	3.5025	3.627	3.2475	3.5038
Average SNRI		2.7488	3.1006	3.9099	3.9080	3.0470

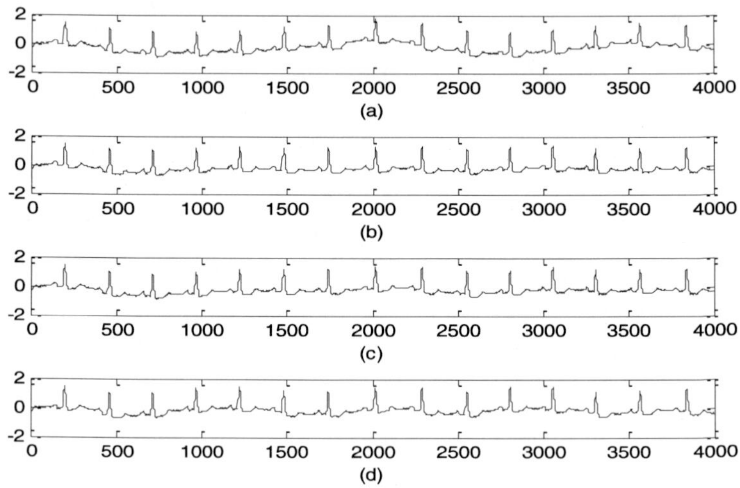

Figure 3.14. Typical filtering results for BW cancellation using sign based LMS algorithm: (a) ECG signal with real BW, (b) recovered signal using SRLMS algorithm, (c) recovered signal using SLMS algorithm, (d) recovered signal using SSLMS algorithm.

The SNRI contrast of the five types of sign based LMS algorithms for BW removal is measured using (3.1) and tabulated in Table 3.7.

Among all the algorithms SRDZLMS gets first place with an average SNRI of 3.8610 dBs, next SRLMF with an average SNRI of 3.0612, SRMLMS achieves 2.9125 dBs, which are more than the SNRI obtained from LMS algorithm. Therefore, using SRA we are achieving better filtering by reduced number of multiplications by an amount equal to the filter length.

Table 3.7. SNRI contrast of sign based adaptive algorithms for the removal of BW

S.No.	Algorithm	Record No. 100	Record No. 105	Record No. 108	Record No. 203	Record No. 228	Average SNRI
1.	SRLMS	2.7786	2.9869	2.0596	2.2602	2.9598	2.4080
2.	SLMS	1.7147	2.5292	1.8447	1.9801	2.4919	2.1121
3.	SSLMS	1.4172	1.8922	1.3945	1.3044	1.8530	1.5722
4.	SRLLMS	1.9374	2.5390	2.5748	2.4937	2.9322	2.4954
5.	SLLMS	1.5840	2.1419	2.0865	2.2099	2.5188	2.1082
6.	SSLLMS	1.2893	1.9074	1.9456	1.7784	1.8028	1.7447
7.	SRDZLMS	4.3811	4.5439	3.6445	3.3224	3.4134	3.8610
8.	SDZLMS	3.1388	2.6654	2.9358	2.8552	3.2965	2.9783
9.	SSDZLMS	2.4317	2.0410	2.4286	2.5653	2.7125	2.4358
10.	SRLMF	3.1714	3.3503	2.9956	2.9690	2.8199	3.0612
11.	SLMF	1.7147	2.5292	1.8447	1.9801	2.4919	2.1121
12.	SSLMF	1.4172	1.8922	1.3945	1.3044	1.8530	1.5722
13.	SRMLMS	2.5190	2.8128	2.9903	3.4246	2.8160	2.9125
14.	SMLMS	2.0219	2.0167	2.2038	2.9682	2.3426	2.3106
15.	SSMLMS	1.9224	1.9918	1.8038	1.9682	1.8297	1.9031

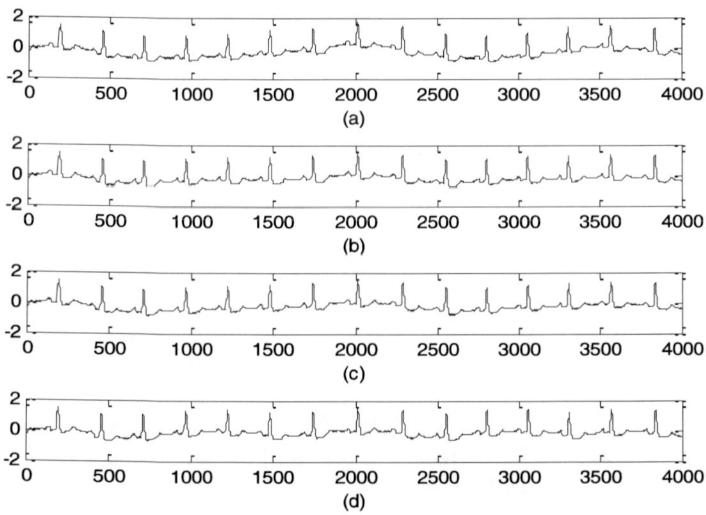

Figure 3.15. Typical filtering results for BW cancellation using sign based LLMS algorithm: (a) ECG signal with real BW, (b) recovered signal using SRLLMS algorithm, (c) recovered signal using SLLMS algorithm, (d) recovered signal using SSLLMS algorithm.

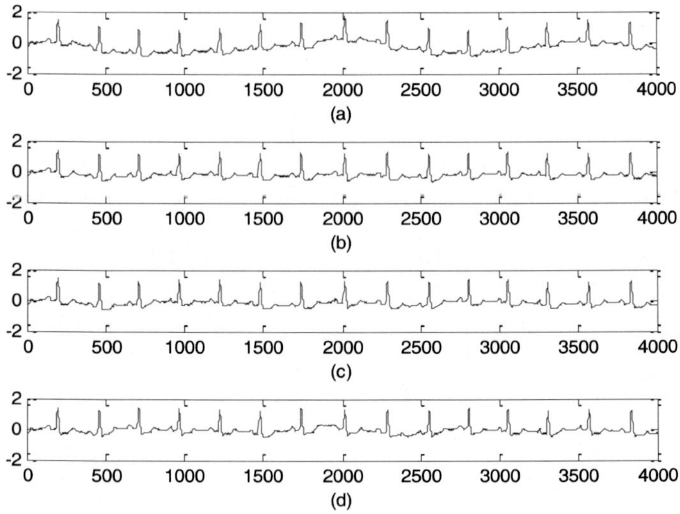

Figure 3.16. Typical filtering results for BW cancellation using sign based DZLMS algorithm: (a) ECG signal with real BW, (b) recovered signal using SRDZLMS algorithm, (c) recovered signal using SDZLMS algorithm, (d) recovered signal using SSDZLMS algorithm.

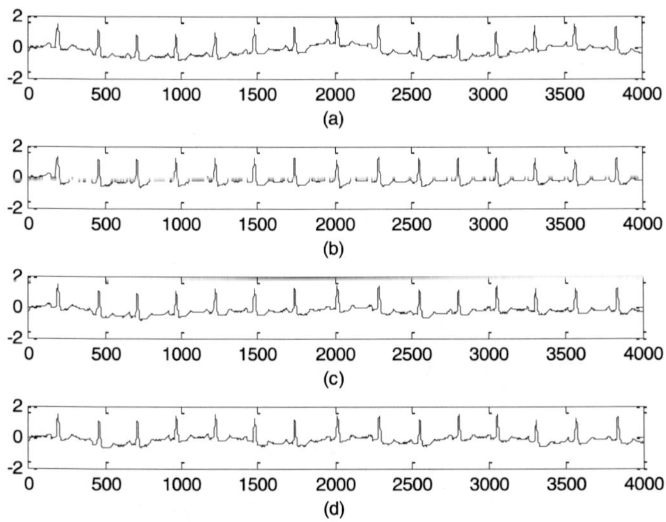

Figure 3.17. Typical filtering results for BW cancellation using sign based LMF algorithm: (a) ECG signal with real BW, (b) recovered signal using SRLMF algorithm, (c) recovered signal using SLMF algorithm, (d) recovered signal using SSLMF algorithm.

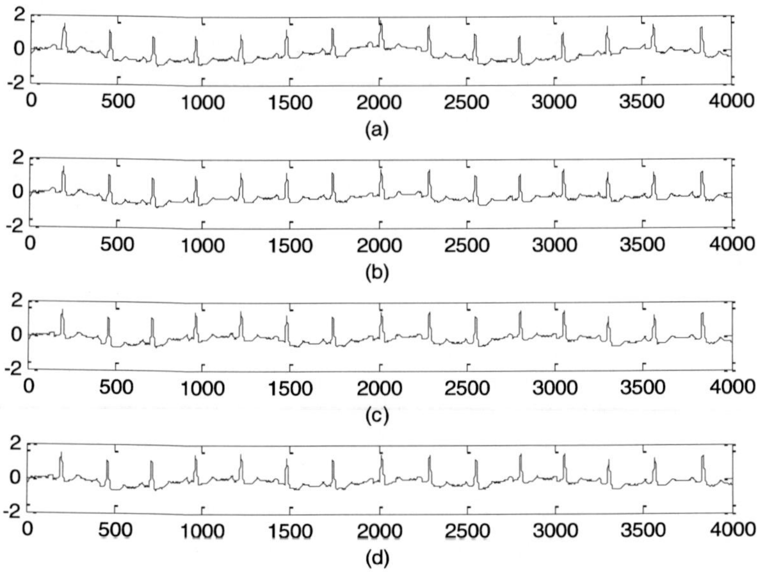

Figure 3.18. Typical filtering results for BW cancellation using sign based MLMS algorithm: (a) ECG signal with real BW, (b) recovered signal using SRMLMS algorithm, (c) recovered signal using SMLMS algorithm, (d) recovered signal using SSMLMS algorithm.

3.9.4. Adaptive Cancellation of Muscle Artefacts

This experiment proves MA cancellation from ECG signals, which is a non- stationary noise cancellation. The input to the filter is ECG signal is contaminated with respiration baseline wander; this is applied to a noise canceller shown in Figure 2.3. The reference signal is a real MA obtained from MIT-BIH Noise Stress Test Database. The MA originally had a sampling frequency of 360Hz and therefore they were anti-alias re-sampled to 128Hz in order to match the sampling rate of the ECG. Various filter structures are implemented using LMS, LLMS, DLMS, LMF and MLMS algorithms. The simulation results for LMS based ANCs are shown in Figure 3.19.

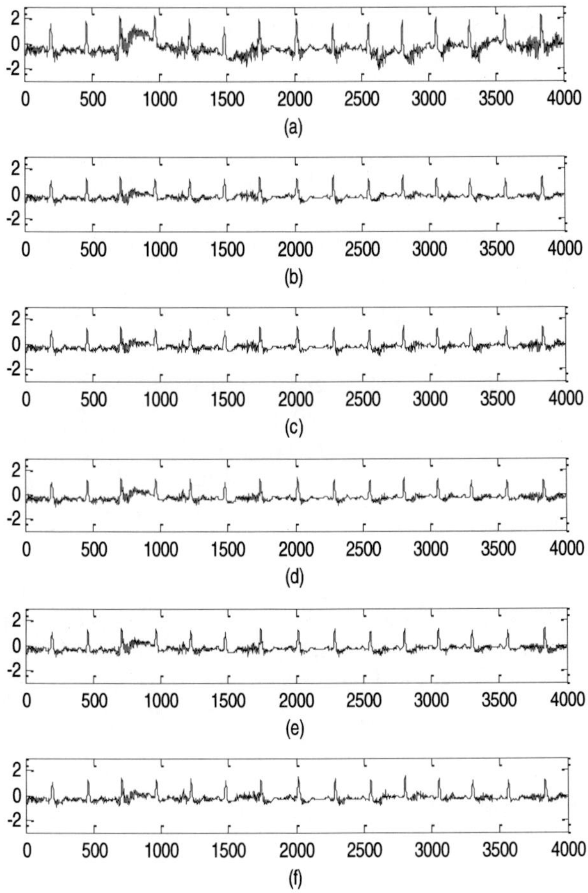

Figure 3.19. Typical filtering results for MA removal using LMS based adaptive filtering techniques: (a) ECG signal with real MA, (b) recovered signal using LMS algorithm, (c) recovered signal using LLMS algorithm, (d) recovered signal using DZLMS algorithm, (e) recovered signal using LMF algorithm, (f) recovered signal using MLMS algorithm.

The SNRI for various filtering methods are measured based on (3.1) and are shown in Table 3.8.

From the table it is clear that LMF effectively filters MA noise, it got an average SNRI of 5.4617 dBs, DZLMS gets 5.4386 dBs, LLMS gets 4.7189 dBs, MLMS get 4.5069 dBs whereas conventional LMS gets 4.6128 dBs. From this it is noticed that the performance of LLMS and MLMS is slightly reduces from LMS. The excess mean square error

(EMSE) and misadjustment (M_{ad}) due to various ANCs in different artefact environments are measured using MATLAB programs based on (2.4), (2.2) and are tabulated in Table 3.12. In evidence with filtering capability of the algorithms, minimum EMSE and M_{ad} are obtained by DZLMS and LMF algorithms.

Table 3.8. SNRI contrast of adaptive algorithms for the removal of MA

S. No	Record No	LMS	LLMS	DZLMS	LMF	MLMS
1.	100	3.5006	3.9336	4.5595	4.7520	3.4635
2.	105	4.9304	5.2895	5.7081	5.9820	4.9736
3.	108	3.9917	4.1581	5.2605	5.5493	3.4621
4.	203	5.1927	5.3423	5.7288	5.5337	5.7719
5.	228	4.7286	4.8713	5.9362	5.4917	4.8636
Average SNRI		4.6128	4.7189	5.4386	5.4617	4.5069

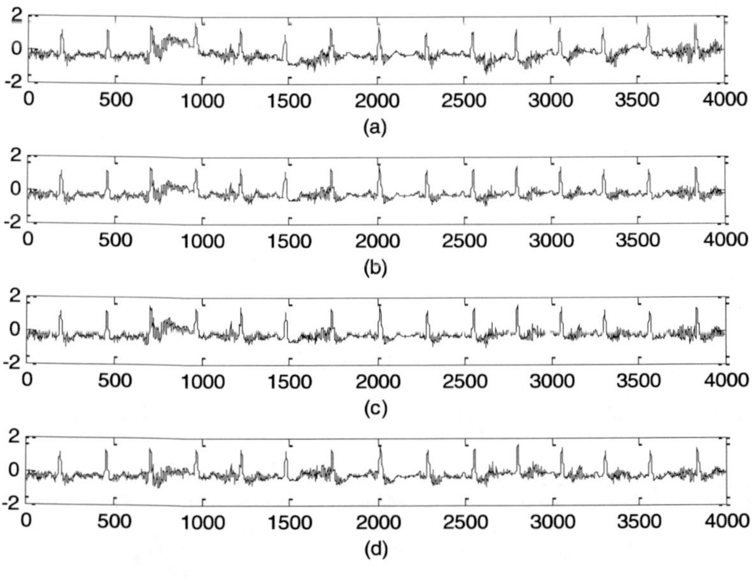

Figure 3.20. Typical filtering results for MA cancellation using sign based LMS algorithm: (a) ECG signal with real MA, (b) recovered signal using SRLMS algorithm, (c) recovered signal using SLMS algorithm, (d) recovered signal using SSLMS algorithm.

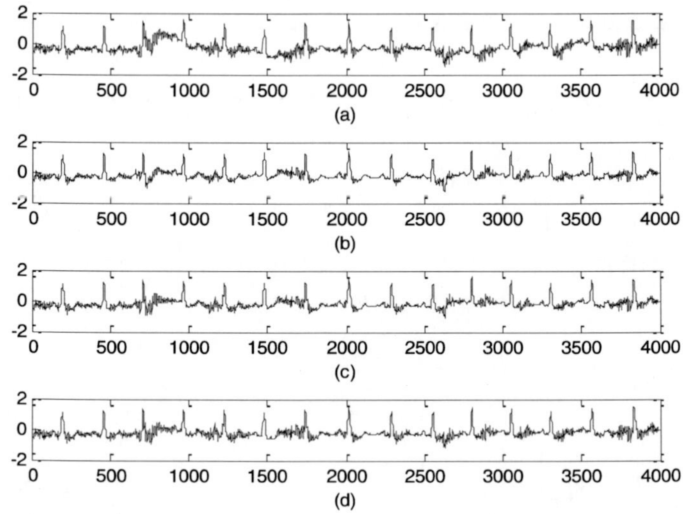

Figure 3.21. Typical filtering results for MA cancellation using sign based LLMS algorithm: (a) ECG signal with real MA, (b) recovered signal using SRLLMS algorithm, (c) recovered signal using SLLMS algorithm, (d) recovered signal using SSLLMS algorithm.

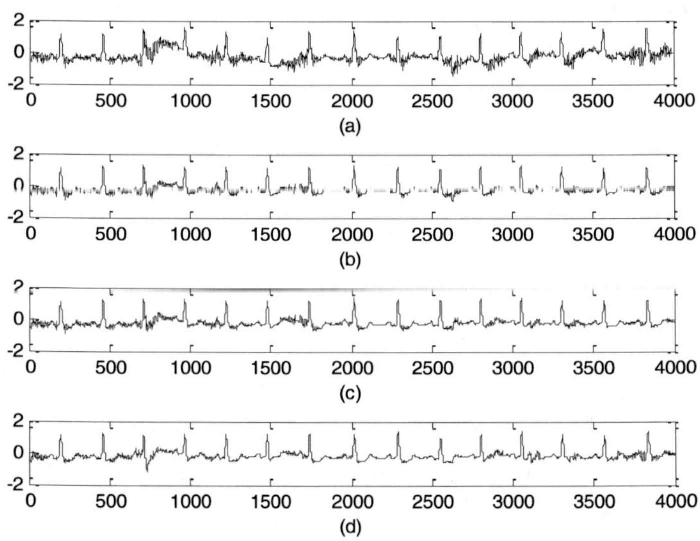

Figure 3.22. Typical filtering results for MA cancellation using sign based DZLMS algorithm: (a) ECG signal with real MA, (b) recovered signal using SRDZLMS algorithm, (c) recovered signal using SDZLMS algorithm, (d) recovered signal using SSDZLMS algorithm.

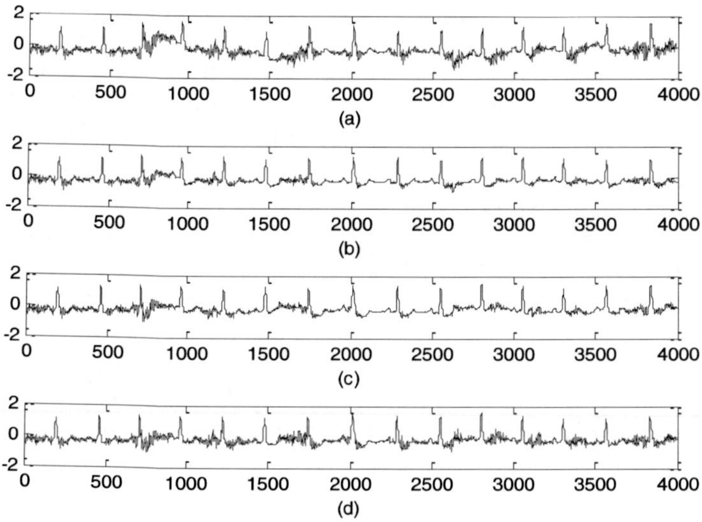

Figure 3.23. Typical filtering results for MA cancellation using sign based LMF algorithm: (a) ECG signal with real MA, (b) recovered signal using SRLMF algorithm, (c) recovered signal using SLMF algorithm, (d) recovered signal using SSLMF algorithm.

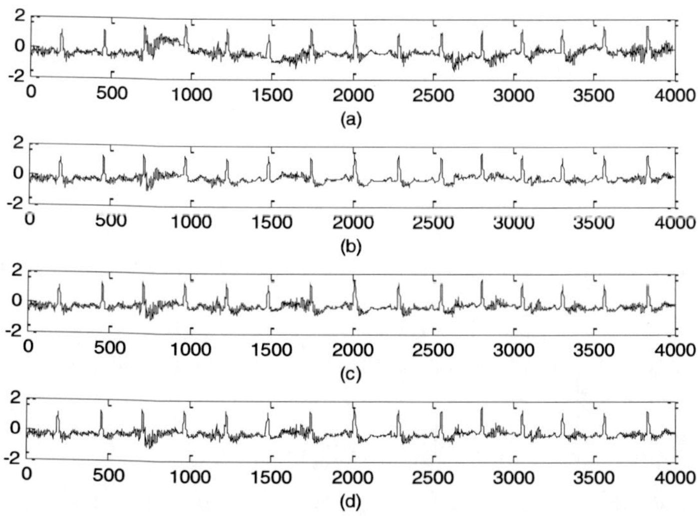

Figure 3.24. Typical filtering results for MA cancellation using sign based MLMS algorithm: (a) ECG signal with real MA, (b) recovered signal using SRMLMS algorithm, (c) recovered signal using SMLMS algorithm, (d) recovered signal using SSMLMS algorithm.

To enjoy the less computational complexity the LMS based adaptive algorithms are combined with signed algorithms and results several algorithms. These are SRLMS, SLMS, SSLMS, SRLLMS, SLLMS, SSLLMS, SRDZLMS, SDZLMS, SSDZLMS, SRLMF, SLMF, SSLMF, SRMLMS, SMLMS and SSMLMS. Using these algorithms various ANCs are developed and tested for the removal of MA. The filtering results are as follows from Figure 3.20 to Figure 3.24.

The SNRI contrast of various sign based LMS algorithms for MA removal is given in Table 3.9. Among all the algorithms SRDZLMS gets first place with an average SNRI of 4.0833 dBs, this is very close to that of conventional LMS algorithm, which is 4.6128 dBs, SRLMF gets 3.7426 dBs, SRMLMS gets 2.9557 dBs, SRLLMS gets 2.5089 dBs.

Table 3.9. SNRI contrast of s sign based adaptive algorithms for the removal of MA

S.No.	Algorithm	Record No. 100	Record No. 105	Record No. 108	Record No. 203	Record No. 228	Average SNRI
1.	SRLMS	2.2715	2.8415	2.4805	3.8436	3.0749	2.9024
2.	SLMS	2.0165	2.5719	2.3044	2.9911	2.8945	2.5556
3.	SSLMS	1.7931	2.2579	2.0441	2.8784	2.2191	2.2385
4.	SRLLMS	2.0564	2.6486	2.3093	2.9698	2.5608	2.5089
5.	SLLMS	1.8001	2.3121	1.6932	1.9954	1.8849	1.9371
6.	SSLLMS	1.3029	2.0996	1.3508	1.9028	1.3767	1.6065
7.	SRDZLMS	5.0356	3.9533	2.5045	4.0761	4.8472	4.0833
8.	SDZLMS	3.4552	3.3313	2.0330	3.5061	3.7485	3.2148
9.	SSDZLMS	2.0846	2.7578	1.7176	2.9625	2.1877	2.3420
10.	SRLMF	4.0952	3.5648	2.6021	4.0081	4.4432	3.7426
11.	SLMF	2.0165	2.5719	2.3044	2.9911	2.8945	2.5556
12.	SSLMF	1.7931	2.2579	2.0441	2.8784	2.2191	2.2385
13.	SRMLMS	2.0386	2.7729	2.3214	4.6840	2.9620	2.9557
14.	SMLMS	1.8393	2.6392	2.2291	3.5966	2.8159	2.6240
15.	SSMLMS	1.7225	2.1048	2.0181	2.9114	2.1977	2.1909

3.9.5. Adaptive Cancellation of Electrode Motion Artefacts

This experiment demonstrates EM cancellation, which is a non-stationary noise cancellation. The input to the filter is ECG signal is contaminated with respiration baseline wander; this is applied to a noise canceller shown in Figure 2.3. The reference signal is a real EM obtained from MIT-BIH Noise Stress Test Database. The EM originally had a sampling frequency of 360Hz and therefore they were anti-alias re-sampled to 128Hz in order to match the sampling rate of the ECG. Various filter structures are implemented using LMS, LLMS, DLMS, LMF and MLMS algorithms.

Table 3.10. SNRI contrast of adaptive algorithms for the removal of EM

S. No	Record No	LMS	LLMS	DZLMS	LMF	MLMS
1.	100	2.7289	2.9187	5.0286	4.6813	4.3705
2.	105	3.9484	4.2460	5.1066	5.1127	4.2589
3.	108	3.0080	3.4475	4.9660	5.2069	3.3894
4.	203	3.3268	3.7481	4.9535	5.7547	3.9291
5.	228	3.6710	3.6723	3.7390	3.7159	3.8203
Average SNRI		3.3366	3.6065	4.7587	4.8943	3.9536

The simulation results for all LMS based ANCs are shown in Figure 3.25. The SNRI for various filtering methods is shown in Table 3.10. From this table it is clear that LMF effectively filters EM noise, it got an average SNRI of 4.8943 dBs, DZLMS gets 4.7587 dBs, MLMS gets 3.9536 dBs and LLMS get 3.6065 dBs whereas conventional LMS gets 3.3366 dBs. From this it is noticed that the performance of LLMS is slightly inferior to that of LMS. The EMSE and M_{ad} due to various ANCs in different artefact environments are calculated using MATLAB programs written based on (2.4) and (2.2) and are tabulated in Table 3.12.

To enjoy the less computational complexity the gradient based adaptive algorithms are combined with signed algorithms and results several algorithms. These are SRLMS, SLMS, SSLMS, SRLLMS,

SLLMS, SSLLMS, SRDZLMS, SDZLMS, SSDZLMS, SRLMF, SLMF, SSLMF, SRMLMS, SMLMS and SSMLMS. Using these algorithms various ANCs are developed and tested for the removal of EM. The filtering results are as follows from Figure 3.26 to Figure3.30.

The SNRI contrast of various sign-based algorithms for EM removal is given in Table 3.11. Among all the algorithms SRDZLMS gets first place with an average SNRI of 4.0097 dBs, SRLMF gets 3.8439 dBs, SRMLMS gets 2.4523 dBs and SRLLMS gets 2.3677 dBs whereas the conventional LMS algorithm gets 2.9024 dBs.

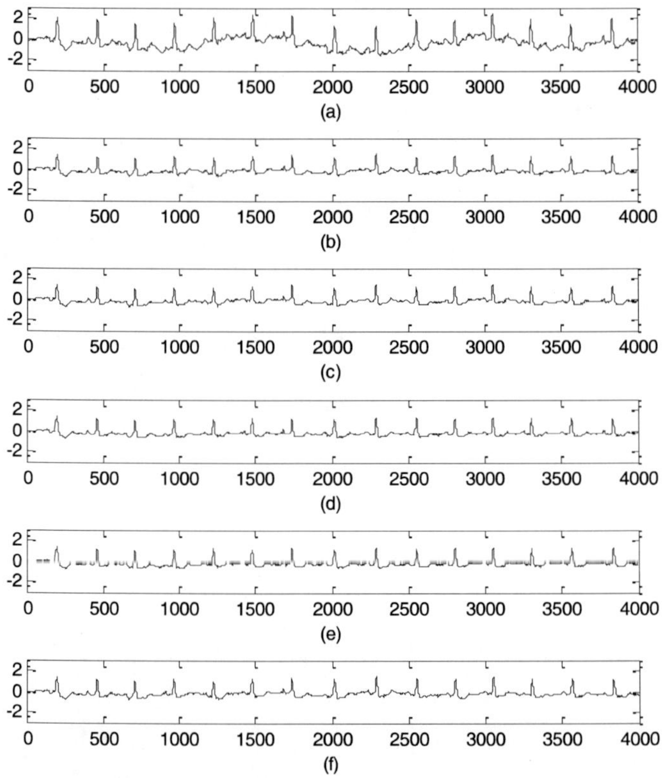

Figure 3.25. Typical filtering results for EM removal using LMS based adaptive filtering techniques: (a) ECG signal with real EM, (b) recovered signal using LMS algorithm, (c) recovered signal using LLMS algorithm, (d) recovered signal using DLMS algorithm, (e) recovered signal using LMF algorithm, (f) recovered signal using MLMS algorithm.

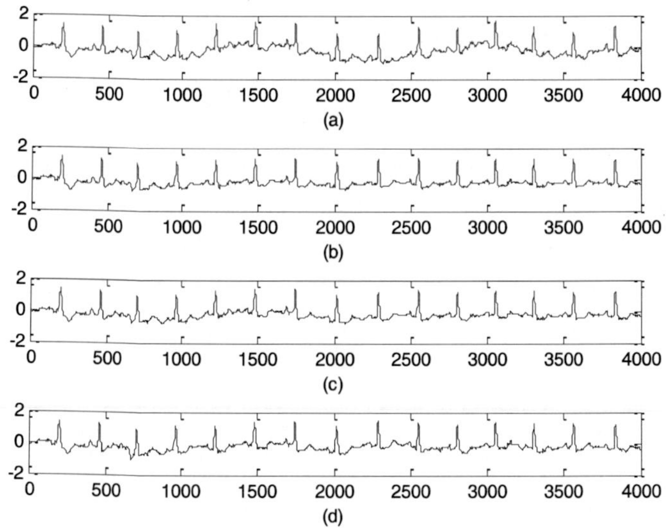

Figure 3.26. Typical filtering results for EM cancellation using sign based LMS algorithm: (a) ECG signal with real EM, (b) recovered signal using SRLMS algorithm, (c) recovered signal using SLMS algorithm, (d) recovered signal using SSLMS algorithm.

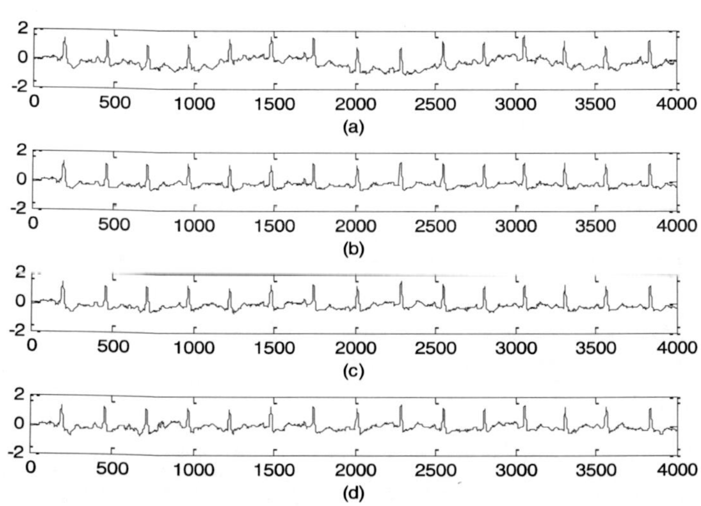

Figure 3.27. Typical filtering results for EM cancellation using sign based LLMS algorithm: (a) ECG signal with real EM, (b) recovered signal using SRLLMS algorithm, (c) recovered signal using SLLMS algorithm, (d) recovered signal using SSLLMS algorithm.

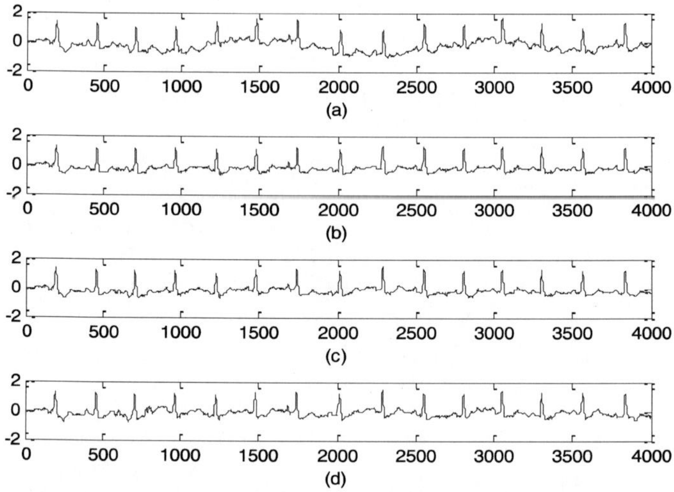

Figure 3.28. Typical filtering results for EM cancellation using sign based DZLMS algorithm: (a) ECG signal with real EM, (b) recovered signal using SRDZLMS algorithm, (c) recovered signal using SDZLMS algorithm, (d) recovered signal using SSDZLMS algorithm.

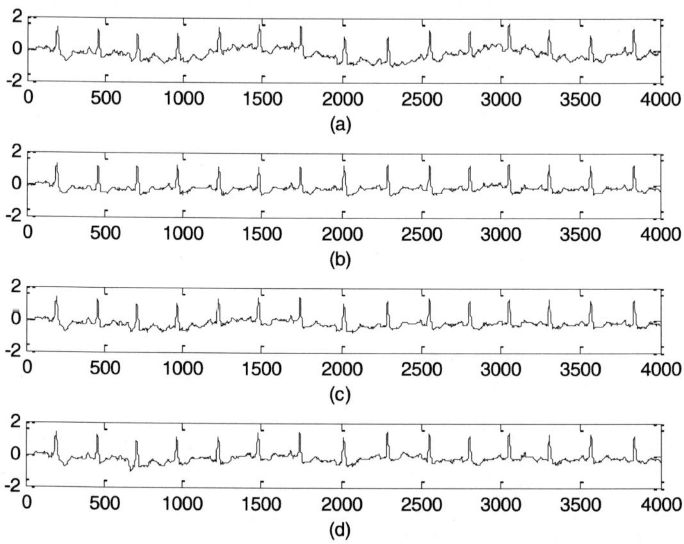

Figure 3.29. Typical filtering results for EM cancellation using sign based LMF algorithm: (a) ECG signal with real EM, (b) recovered signal using SRLMF algorithm, (c) recovered signal using SLMF algorithm, (d) recovered signal using SSLMF algorithm.

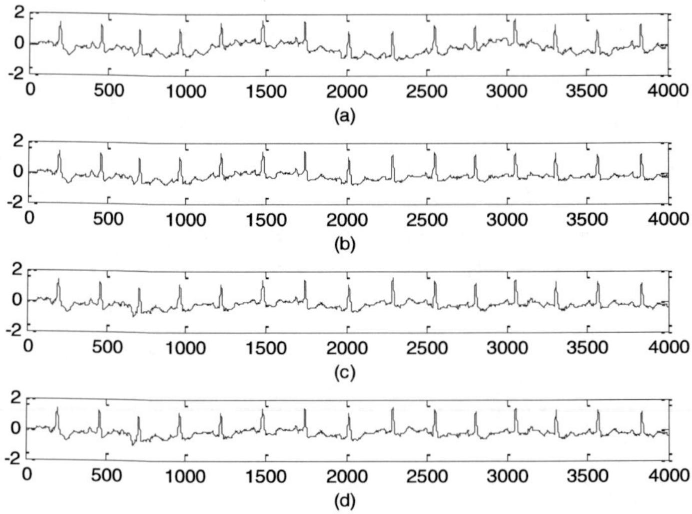

Figure 3.30. Typical filtering results for EM cancellation using sign based MLMS algorithm: (a) ECG signal with real EM, (b) recovered signal using SRMLMS algorithm, (c) recovered signal using SMLMS algorithm, (d) recovered signal using SSMLMS algorithm

Table 3.11. SNRI contrast of sign based adaptive algorithms for the removal of EM

S.No.	Algorithm	Record No. 100	Record No. 105	Record No. 108	Record No. 203	Record No. 228	Average SNRI
1.	SRLMS	1.8702	3.1866	2.2370	2.8073	2.7846	**2.5771**
2.	SLMS	1.7412	2.9397	1.9640	2.6902	2.3351	**2.3340**
3.	SSLMS	1.4392	2.7773	1.6241	2.1847	2.2325	**2.0515**
4.	SRLLMS	1.8109	2.8020	2.2574	2.5070	2.4590	**2.3672**
5.	SLLMS	1.6360	2.3306	1.9364	1.9895	2.3984	**2.0581**
6.	SSLLMS	1.2818	2.0071	1.7794	1.8701	1.9845	**1.7845**
7.	SRDZLMS	5.0884	4.8700	2.7826	3.1874	4.1245	**4.0097**
8.	SDZLMS	3.0861	2.7243	1.9261	2.2935	2.6389	**2.5337**
9.	SSDZLMS	0.9226	1.3027	1.2013	1.4425	1.1990	**1.3718**
10.	SRLMF	9.5324	4.9500	2.8202	3.4293	3.4879	**3.8439**
11.	SLMF	1.7412	2.9397	1.9640	2.6902	2.3351	**2.3340**
12.	SSLMF	1.4392	2.7773	1.6241	2.1847	2.2325	**2.0515**
13.	SRMLMS	1.8370	2.8492	2.2210	2.7194	2.6349	**2.4523**
14.	SMLMS	1.1577	2.4389	1.9585	2.3858	2.3420	**2.0565**
15.	SSMLMS	1.1247	2.2001	1.9090	1.8225	2.0204	**1.8153**

Table 3.12. A comparison of EMSE and M_{ad} for various artifacts using LMS and its variant algorithms

Noise Type	R. No	LMS		LLMS		DZLMS		LMF		MLMS	
		EMSE	M_{ad}	EMSE	M_{ad}	EMSE	M_{ad}	EMSE	M_{ad}	EMSE	M_{ad}
PLI	100	-19.9894	0.0761	-26.0233	0.0190	-21.4043	0.0549	-20.7950	0.0632	-24.9926	0.0191
	105	-21.8298	0.0460	-27.1402	0.0135	-22.1757	0.0425	-23.8734	0.0287	-25.7989	0.0192
	108	-20.5036	0.0744	-24.7714	0.0279	-21.5962	0.0579	-22.0829	0.0518	-23.3700	0.0306
	203	-21.5394	0.0134	-27.2784	0.0071	-22.8202	0.0199	-25.6271	0.0083	-26.7658	0.0151
	228	-21.5227	0.0725	-25.7233	0.0276	-21.9834	0.0652	-23.3712	0.0376	-24.9245	0.0263
	Avg	**-21.0769**	**0.0564**	**-26.1873**	**0.0190**	**-21.9959**	**0.0480**	**-23.1499**	**0.0379**	**-25.1703**	**0.0220**
BW	100	-11.1457	0.5829	-11.8386	0.4969	-17.2048	0.1444	-15.7115	0.2565	-11.2754	0.5658
	105	-11.4418	0.5030	-12.8057	0.3675	-13.6397	0.3033	-12.7590	0.3714	-11.5310	0.4928
	108	-11.4700	0.5960	-12.2577	0.4971	-12.3672	0.6102	-12.2379	0.4994	-11.6089	0.5772
	203	-8.9635	0.4842	-10.2557	0.3596	-11.0885	0.4705	-10.8838	0.4932	-9.0180	0.4782
	228	-12.6204	0.5630	-13.5362	0.4559	-17.1546	0.1493	-17.1185	0.1998	-12.7328	0.5486
	Avg	**-11.1282**	**0.5458**	**-12.1387**	**0.4354**	**-14.2909**	**0.3355**	**-13.7421**	**0.3640**	**-11.2332**	**0.5325**
MA	100	-12.1110	0.4667	-12.1897	0.4584	-16.0276	0.1894	-14.9272	0.2440	-11.5792	0.5275
	105	-12.4097	0.4025	-12.4682	0.3972	-14.8754	0.2282	-14.0851	0.2737	-12.2046	0.4220
	108	-11.7569	0.5579	-11.8251	0.5492	-13.1811	0.4019	-13.0987	0.4096	-11.4107	0.5610
	203	-11.1118	0.8090	-11.7505	0.7078	-17.4823	0.3660	-14.1892	0.4815	-10.8163	0.9305
	228	-13.8287	0.4262	-13.9327	0.4162	-20.4342	0.0931	-18.3396	0.1509	-13.0058	0.6092
	Avg	**-12.3426**	**0.5324**	**-12.4332**	**0.5057**	**-16.4001**	**0.2557**	**-14.9279**	**0.3119**	**-11.8033**	**0.6100**
EM	100	-10.7955	0.6319	-10.8499	0.6240	-15.0222	0.3551	-15.2980	0.2285	-11.5703	0.5286
	105	-10.7225	0.5936	-10.7470	0.5903	-13.0016	0.4513	-14.1302	0.4293	-11.7866	0.4946
	108	-10.9025	0.6792	-10.9700	0.6687	-12.9328	0.5844	-13.5803	0.4710	-11.6255	0.5750
	203	-8.2407	0.5719	-8.2617	0.5692	-10.1697	0.3814	-11.0769	0.3539	-9.1318	0.4683
	228	-12.3952	0.5929	-12.4630	0.5837	-15.7605	0.2878	-15.9061	0.2631	-13.2715	0.4846
	Avg	**-10.6112**	**0.6139**	**-10.6583**	**0.6071**	**-13.3773**	**0.4120**	**-13.9983**	**0.3491**	**-11.4771**	**0.5102**

From Table 3.12, it is clear that for the PLI removal LLMS gets lowest EMSE, next MLMS gets, similarly the M_{ad} is for LLMS is minimum among all five algorithms and next place goes to MLMS. In the BW removal DZLMS achieves lower EMSE, next LMF achieves lower EMSE and similarly the M_{ad} is lower for these two algorithms. For the MA and EM removal also DZLMS and LMF exhibits minimum EMSE and $M_{ad.}$

3.10. Conclusion

In this chapter, we have developed weight update variants of LMS based adaptive algorithms. Using these algorithms various ANCs are developed for the denoising of ECG signals. To achieve fast data transmission rate, it is desirable to reduce the computational complexity. This can be done by clipping either the estimation error or the input data. The signed algorithms are derived based on this clipping; the three versions of signed algorithms are utilized here. Now we have extended the LMS based adaptive algorithms to the three versions of sign based adaptive algorithms. Totally twenty adaptive noise cancellers are developed and tested on ECG signals. These are LMS, LLMS, DZLMS, LMF and MLMS algorithms and their fifteen sign-based algorithms i.e., SRLMS, SLMS, SSLMS, SRLLMS, SLLMS, SSLMS, SRDZLMS, SDZLMS, SSDZLMS, SRLMF, SLMF, SSLMF, SRMLMS, SMLMS and SSMLMS algorithms. Thc LMS algorithm is implcmented for standardization purpose. To evaluate the performance of the various ANCs we have plotted the convergence characteristics, computational complexity, SNRI, EMSE and M_{ad} are calculated. Among the five LMS based algorithms DZLMS and LMF algorithms performs better in the non-stationary noise removal. Among the sign-based versions sign regressor version of algorithms performs better. All the remaining SA and SSA based ANCs are slightly inferior to their LMS counterpart. The Sign-sign version of LMS based algorithms is free from multiplications and entire weight updating can be carried with the help of addition with sign check operations. In this chapter twenty adaptive algorithm-based ANCs are developed using MATLAB for four types of noises along with channel noise. Among the twenty algorithms SRLMS, DZSRLMS based ANCs are considered for development on digital signal processor as they perform better in terms of SNRI and computational complexity.

Chapter 4

NORMALIZATION BASED REALIZATION OF ADAPTIVE FILTERING TECHNIQUES FOR THE REMOVAL OF NOISE IN THE ECG SIGNALS

4.1. INTRODUCTION

In clinical situations we need to remove artefacts from ECG signals for the extraction of high-resolution signals. In order to achieve fast convergence and good filtering capability, in this Chapter we introduce normalization-based ANCs and their sign-based versions to reduce computational burden. The familiar LMS algorithm has wide applications because of its simplicity and robustness. The LMS filter requires a priori knowledge of the input power level to select the step size parameter for stability and convergence. Since the input power level is usually one of the statistically unknowns, it is normally estimated from the data prior to beginning the adaptation process. But in practical situations it suffers with two drawbacks. These can be well explained from its weight recursion. By observing the weight update recursion of LMS algorithm given by (2.17) it is clear that the input data vector is directly proportional to the weight update mechanism. Another one is the step size is fixed. In practice an algorithm has to be designed such that, it has to tackle both strong and weak signals. Hence depending upon the filter input and output fluctuations, the tap coefficients should be adjusted accordingly. Therefore, when the input data vector is large, LMS algorithm suffers from a gradient noise amplification problem. To avoid this problem normalized LMS (NLMS) can be used. By doing so the adjustment applied to filter weight vector coefficient is normalized with respect to squared Eclidian norm of the input vector at each iteration.

Table 4.1. Summary of algorithms used in Chapter 4

S. No	Acronym	Name	Advantage
1.	NLMS	Normalized Least Mean Square	Fast convergence, avoids gradient noise amplification problem
2.	ENLMS	Error nonlinear least mean square	Fast convergence, minimizes signal distortion
3.	NSRLMS	Normalized sign regressor least mean square	Fast convergence, avoids gradient noise amplification problem, only one multiplication needed to compute the recursion
4.	NSLMS	Normalized sign least mean square	Fast convergence, avoids gradient noise amplification problem, it requires L MACs
5.	NSSLMS	Normalized sign sign least mean square	Fast convergence, avoids gradient noise amplification problem, zero multiplications required, enter recursion is computed with addition with sign check operation
6.	ENSRLMS	Error nonlinear sign regressor least mean square	Fast convergence, minimizes signal distortion, only one multiplication needed to compute the recursion
7.	ENSLMS	Error nonlinear sign least mean square	Fast convergence, minimizes signal distortion, it requires L MACs
8.	ENSSLMS	Error nonlinear sign sign least mean square	Fast convergence, minimizes signal distortion, zero multiplications required, enter recursion is computed with addition with sign check operation

Because of the fixed step size, the convergence speed is low in conventional LMS algorithm. In order to increase the convergence speed of the LMS filter without using estimates of the input signal correlation matrix, a variable convergence factor is the best remedy. Because of normalization, the step size varies iteratively; this step size is proportional to the inverse of the total expected energy of the instantaneous values of the coefficients of the input data vector. The normalized LMS algorithm usually converges faster than the LMS algorithm, since it utilizes a variable convergence factor aiming at the minimization of the instantaneous output error [91, 113, 114]. Several contributions on NLMS are given in [92, 95]. Other strategies for varying the step size are reported in [81, 85]. The summary of algorithms used in this chapter is given in Table 4.1.

4.2. Normalized Adaptive Algorithms

The normalized version LMS over comes the two drawbacks discussed above by considering the variation in the signal level at the filter output and selecting the normalized step size parameter that results in a stable as well as fast converging algorithm. In the normalization version of the LMS algorithm the correlation between the error and the reference input is normalized by a factor equal to the squared norm. Here we consider two types of normalizations, namely data normalization and error normalization. These results Normalized LMS (NLMS) algorithm and Error Nonlinear LMS or Error Normalized LMS (ENLMS) algorithm respectively, detailed as follows.

4.2.1. The Normalized LMS Algorithm

NLMS algorithm is another class of adaptive algorithm used to train the coefficients of the adaptive filter. One of the problems in design and implementation of the LMS adaptive filter is the selection of the step size. For the stationary process the LMS algorithm converges in the mean if $0 < \mu < \frac{2}{\lambda_{max}}$ and converges in the mean square if $0 < \mu < \frac{2}{tr(R_x)}$, however, since the R_x is generally unknown then either, λ_{max} or R_x, must be estimated in order to use these bounds.

The bound on the step size for mean-square convergence:

$$0 < \mu < \frac{2}{\boldsymbol{x}^T(n)\boldsymbol{x}(n)}$$

more over the upper bound is given as

$$\mu(n) = \frac{\mu}{\boldsymbol{x}^T(n)\boldsymbol{x}(n)} = \frac{\mu}{||\boldsymbol{x}(n)||2} \tag{4.1}$$

In overcoming the gradient noise amplification problem associated with the conventional LMS filter, the normalized LMS filter introduces a problem of its own, namely the tap input vector **x**(n) is small, numerical difficulties may arise because then we have to divide by a small value for the squared norm. To overcome this problem, we modify the above recursion by adding a small positive constant ε. The parameter ε is set to avoid denominator being too small and step size parameter is too big.

Now the step size parameter is written as,

$$\mu(n) = \frac{\mu}{\varepsilon + ||\boldsymbol{x}(n)||2} \tag{4.2}$$

where $\mu(n)$ is a normalized step size with $0 < \mu < 2$. Replacing μ in the LMS weight vector update equation with $\mu(n)$ leads to the NLMS, which is given as

$$\boldsymbol{w}(n+1) = \boldsymbol{w}(n) + \frac{\mu}{||\boldsymbol{x}(n)||2} e(n)\boldsymbol{x}(n) \tag{4.3}$$

In the LMS algorithm, the correction that is applied $\mathbf{w}(n)$ is proportional to the input vector $\mathbf{x}(n)$ is large, the LMS algorithm experiences a problem with gradient noise amplification. With the normalization of the LMS step size by $||\boldsymbol{x}(n)||^2$ in the NLMS algorithm, however, this noise amplification problem is diminished. Although the

NLMS algorithm bypasses the problem of noise amplification, we are now faced with a similar problem that occur when $||\boldsymbol{x}(n)||$ becomes too small. An alternative is to use the following modification to the NLMS algorithm:

$$\boldsymbol{w}(n + 1) = \boldsymbol{w}(n) + \frac{\mu}{\varepsilon + ||x(n)||2} e(n)\boldsymbol{x}(n) \tag{4.4}$$

Comparing (2.17) and (4.4), the update equation of NLMS is a scaled version of that of LMS algorithm. The size of the change to weight vector **w**(n) is therefore be in inversely proportional to the norm of data vector **x**(n). The data vector **x**(n) with a large norm will generally lead to a small change to **w**(n) than a vector with a smaller norm. This normalization results smaller step size values than conventional LMS. The normalized algorithm usually converges faster than the LMS algorithm, since it utilizes a variable convergence factor aiming at the minimization of the instantaneous output error [96].

Hence NLMS is applicable to very high-speed application such as biotelemetry. The step size parameter μ of this algorithm is independent of the input signal power. But this algorithm required more computation to evaluate the normalization term $||\boldsymbol{x}(n)||^2$. At the same time NLMS requires less a priori information than LMS. Thus, the resulting mean-square error of NLMS is larger than that of LMS.

4.2.2. The Error Nonlinear LMS (ENLMS) Algorithm

Instead of using instantaneous data vector for normalization squared norm of the error vector can be used. The length of the error vector is the instantaneous number of iterations. Because the step size is normalized with reference to error this algorithm is called as ENLMS algorithm. In the ENLMS algorithm the time-varying step-size is inversely proportional to the squared norm of the error vector rather than the input data vector as in the NLMS. This algorithm provides significant improvements in minimizing signal distortion [115]. The advantage of the ENLMS algorithm is that the step size can be chosen independent of the input signal power and the number of tap weights. Hence the ENLMS algorithm has a convergence rate and a steady state error better than LMS algorithm.

Thus, the weight update equation of the ENLMS algorithm becomes

$$\boldsymbol{w}(n+1) = \boldsymbol{w}(n) + \frac{\mu}{\varepsilon + \|e(n)\|^2} e(n)\boldsymbol{x}(n) \tag{4.5}$$

where

$$\|e(n)\|^2 = \sum_{k=0}^{N-1} |e(n-k)|^2 \tag{4.6}$$

is the squared norm of the error, $e(n)$, estimated over its entire updated length n. As in (4.4), ε is added in (4.5) to prevent instability of the algorithm if $\|e(n)\|^2$ is too small.

The EN-LMS algorithm may be considered as a variable step-size algorithm in which the fixed step-size μ in the conventional LMS algorithms is replaced by a variable step-size $\beta(n)$, where $\beta(n)$ is given by:

$$\beta(n) = \frac{\mu}{\varepsilon + \|e(n)\|^2} \tag{4.7}$$

The fixed parameter μ is appropriately chosen to achieve the best trade-off between rate of convergence and low final mean-square error. $\|e(n)\|^2$ in (4.7) is an increasing function of the iteration number, n, and thus, $\beta(n)$ is a decreasing function of n.

Compared with other normalized algorithms, the ENLMS algorithm requires a small number of computations. To compute (4.6) with minimum computational complexity, the error value produced in the first iteration is squared and stored. The error value in the second iteration is squared and added to the previous stored value. Then, the result is stored in order to be used in the next iteration, and so on. On the other hand some additional computations are required to compute $\beta(n)$.

4.3. Extension to Sign Based Realizations of NLMS Algorithm

Less computational complexity of the adaptive filter is highly desirable in biotelemetry applications. This reduction generally obtainable by clipping either the input data or estimation error. The algorithms based on clipping of error or data are presented in section 3.6.1, these are SRA, SA and SSA. The combination of these three simplified algorithms with normalized algorithms provides fast convergence and reduced computational complexity.

Among the adaptive algorithms discussed above, the SRA, SA and SSA have a convergence rate and a steady-state error that is slightly inferior to those of the LMS algorithm for the same parameter setting. But, the computational complexity of these algorithms is much less compared to the LMS algorithm. The advantage of the NLMS algorithm is that the step size can be chosen independent of the input signal power and the number of tap weights. Hence the NLMS algorithm has a convergence rate and a steady state error better than LMS algorithm. On the other hand, some additional computations are required to compute $\mu(n)$. In order to cope up with both the complexity and convergence issues without any restrictive tradeoff, we propose normalized sign-based algorithms such as normalized signed regressor LMS (NSRLMS) algorithm, normalized sign LMS (NSLMS) algorithm and normalized sign–sign LMS (NSSLMS) algorithm for the removal of noise from ECG signal.

4.3.1. Normalized Sign Regressor LMS (NSRLMS) Algorithm

The SRA has a convergence rate and a steady-state error that are only slightly inferior to those of the LMS algorithm for the same parameter setting. Bershad [116] compares the convergence rate of the SRA to that of the LMS algorithm to show that the SRA converges slower than the LMS algorithm by a factor of "only" $\Pi / 2$ for the same steady-state error.

Eweda [98] derives stability conditions and convergence rate of the SRA. If certain stability conditions are satisfied, the SRA could replace the LMS algorithm in some applications, significantly reducing the computing time.

By combining (4.4) and (3.10) the weight update recursion for NSRLMS can be written as,

$$\boldsymbol{w}(n + 1) = \boldsymbol{w}(n) + \mu(n)e(n)Sign\{\boldsymbol{x}(n)\} \tag{4.8}$$

Normalized signed regressor LMS algorithm is a counter part of the NLMS algorithm; this is derived from SRA, where the normalizing factor for the SRA equals the absolute values of the input signal vector components. Here no multiplication operation is required to compute the normalization factor. NSRLMS enjoys the advantages of both SRA and NLMS algorithm. Due to the presence of normalizing factor, the steady state error does not depend on the reference input signal power. However, the steady state error depends on the number of taps, the dependence decreases as the number of taps increases [99], the mean square error (MSE) in the steady state is reported that it is greater than that of NLMS by only 2dB for the same value of the step size when the number of taps is sufficiently large. The behavior of the NSRLMS is heavily input dependent and that there are inputs for which the LMS/NLMS is stable while the NSRLMS is unstable. This is a disadvantage of the NSRLMS with respect to NSLMS, since the latter is more stable than the LMS / NLMS algorithm. However, such a stability problem with NSRLMS when the ANC input is Gaussian, such as in the case of biomedical signals processing. With such input the performance of the NSRLMS is superior to that of NSLMS.

4.3.2. Normalized Sign LMS (NSLMS) Algorithm

The sign algorithm takes the signum of the error signal. This algorithm is particularly attractive for its assured convergence in a disturbance and ease of implementation. The SA converges much slower than the LMS algorithm for the same steady state error. The combination of SA and

NLMS enjoys the benefits of both less complexity and fast convergence. Using (4.4) and (3.13) the weight update recursion for NSLMS can be written as,

$$\boldsymbol{w}(n+1) = \boldsymbol{w}(n) + \mu(n)\, Sign\,\{e(n)\}\boldsymbol{x}(n) \tag{4.9}$$

4.3.3. Normalized Sign Sign LMS (NSSLMS) Algorithm

Further simplification of the sign algorithm is sign-sign algorithm. Here the signum of the reference input is used in addition to the signum of error signal. Thus, this requires only one-bit multiplication. Similar to NSRLMS and NSLMS, NSSLSM can be obtained by combining SSA and NLMS algorithm. Using (4.4) and (3.14) the recursion for NSSLMS can be written as,

$$\boldsymbol{w}(n+1) = \boldsymbol{w}(n) + \mu(n)\, Sign\,\{e(n)\}Sign\{\boldsymbol{x}(n)\} \tag{4.10}$$

4.4. Extension to Sign Based Realizations of ENLMS Algorithm

In order to cope up with both the complexity and convergence issues without any restrictive tradeoff we propose various sign based adaptive structures using ENLMS algorithm. These are Error nonlinear signed regressor LMS (ENSRLMS) algorithm, Error nonlinear sign LMS (ENSLMS) algorithm and Error nonlinear sign-sign LMS (ENSSLMS) algorithm. These algorithms enjoy less computational complexity because of the sign present in the algorithm and good filtering capability because of the normalized term.

4.4.1. Error Nonlinear Signed Regressor LMS (ENSRLMS) Algorithm

The ENSRLMS can be obtained by clipping the input date in ENLMS. Using (4.4) the weight recursion for ENSRLMS is written as,

$$\boldsymbol{w}(n+1) = \boldsymbol{w}(n) + \beta(n)e(n)Sign\{\boldsymbol{x}(n)\} \tag{4.11}$$

where the clipped version of input data $sign\{\boldsymbol{x}(n)\}$ is given by (3.11).

4.4.2. Error Nonlinear Sign LMS (ENSLMS) Algorithm

This version of ENLMS can be obtained by clipping the error. In other words, ENSLMS is similar to SLMS given in (3.13) except that the fixed step μ is replaced by a variable step size $\beta(n)$ as given in (4.7).

The weight update relation for this is written as,

$$\boldsymbol{w}(n+1) = \boldsymbol{w}(n) + \beta(n)Sign\{e(n)\}\,\boldsymbol{x}(n) \tag{4.12}$$

4.4.3. Error Nonlinear Sign Sign LMS (ENSSLMS) Algorithm

This is a version of ENLMS in which both data and error are clipped. The weight update recursion is a combination of (4.5) and (3.14), it can be written as,

$$\boldsymbol{w}(n+1) = \boldsymbol{w}(n) + \beta(n)Sign\{e(n)\}Sign\{\boldsymbol{x}(n)\} \tag{4.13}$$

Because of the sign on both data side and error side this algorithm is free from multiplications.

4.5. Computational Complexity Issues

As the sign-based algorithms are largely free from the MAC operations, the proposed schemes provide elegant means to remove the noise from the ECG signal. Table 4.2 provides comparative account of different commonly used algorithms and the proposed algorithm in terms of number of operations required. Among all the algorithms the NLMS is more complex, it requires 2L + 1 MACs and 1 division operations to implement the weight updating (4.6) on DSP processor. Similarly, ENLMS also requires 2L + 1 MACs and 1 division.

The NSSLMS algorithm, which is the combination of SSLMS and NLMS is very much suitable as this algorithm requires L shift, L ASC operations in case of block-based realization or if we choose the value of $\mu(n)$ as a power of 2. Note that ASC and shift operations require less logic circuitry when compared with MAC operations.

Table 4.2. Computational complexity comparison for normalized adaptive algorithms

S. No.	Algorithm	MACs	ASC	Divisions
1.	NLMS	2L + 1	Nil	1
2.	ENLMS	2L + 1	Nil	1
3.	NSRLMS	1	Nil	1
4.	NSLMS	L	Nil	1
5.	NSSLMS	Nil	L	1
6.	ENSRLMS	1	Nil	1
7.	ENSLMS	L	Nil	1
8.	ENSSLMS	Nil	L	1

Similarly, ENSSLMS requires L ASC operations, L shifts and 1 division. From the Table 4.2 it is also clear that the number of computations required for the proposed NSRLMS and ENSRLMS is independent of filter length. NSRLMS and ENSSLMS require only one MAC operation and one division. Whereas NSLMS and ENSLMS requires L MACs and 1 division, among all sign based normalized algorithms discussed in this chapter NSLMS and ENSLMS are complex. Using a technique called distributed arithmetic (DA) we can compute the norm factor with zero multiplications [117].

4.6. CONVERGENCE ANALYSIS

The convergence curves for NLMS algorithm and its signed based algorithms is shown in Figure 4.1, that for ENLMS and its sign-based realizations is shown in Figure 4.2. These curves are obtained during the adaptive power line interference cancellation using various ANCs individually with an adaptive filter of length 5, random variance of 0.01 and step size 0.01. Comparing the characteristics of normalized algorithms with conventional LMS algorithm (shown in Figure 3.1) it is clear that normalized algorithms converges fast. It is also clear that sign based NSLMS, ENSLMS and sign-sign based NSSLMS, ENSSLMS algorithms exhibits slower convergence due to the residual noise component because of the sign present in the algorithm.

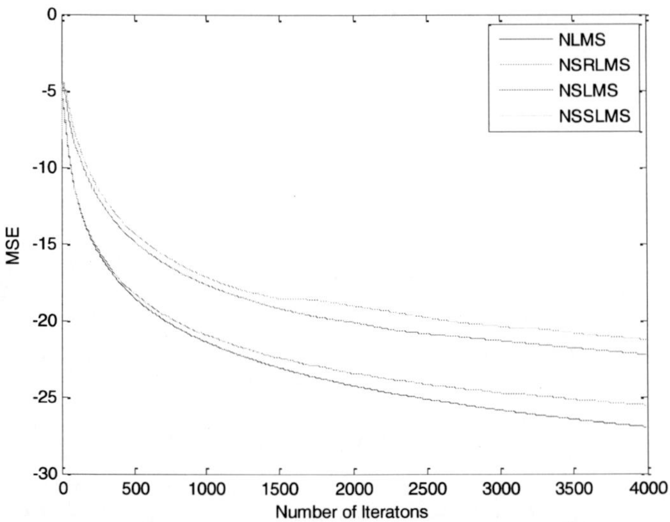

Figure 4.1. Convergence curves of NLMS and its sign-based realizations.

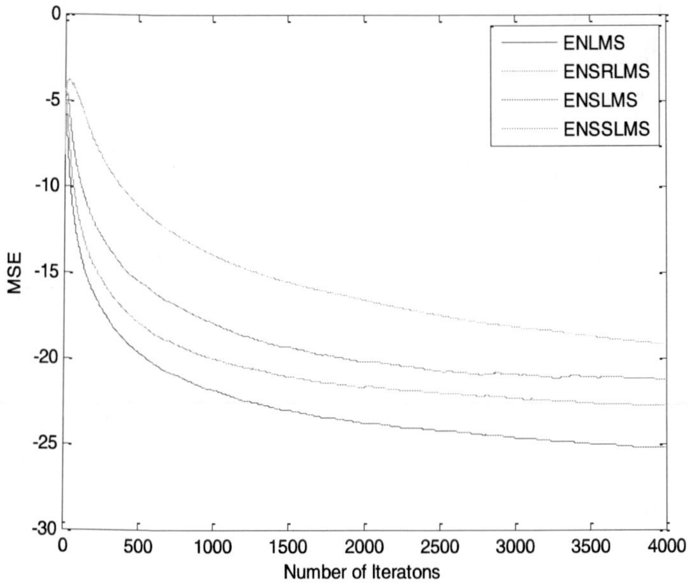

Figure 4.2. Convergence curves of ENLMS and its sign-based realizations.

4.7. RESULTS AND DISCUSSIONS

To test the ability of the normalized adaptive algorithms and their sign-based realizations discussed in this chapter we performed various experiments on real ECG signals with a wide variety of wave morphologies. We used the benchmark MIT-BIH arrhythmia database ECG records for our work [110, 112, 161, 162]. The MIT-BIH Arrhythmia Database contains 48 half-hour excerpts of two-channel ambulatory ECG recordings, obtained from 47 subjects studied by the BIH Arrhythmia Laboratory ages 23 years to 89 years. Twenty-three recordings were chosen at random from a set of 4000, 24-hour ambulatory ECG recordings collected from a mixed population of inpatients (about 60%) and outpatients (about 40%) at Boston's Beth Israel Hospital; the remaining 25 recordings were selected from the same set to include less common but clinically significant arrhythmias that would not be well-represented in a small random sample.

The ECG recordings were made using Del Mar Avionics model 445 two-channel reel-to-reel Holter recorders, and the analog signals were recreated for digitization using a Del Mar Avionics model 660 play-back unit. The computers used for digitization were designed and built in our laboratory, including the tape-drive controllers and the analog-to-digital converter (ADC) interfaces; they used then state-of-the-art 1 MHz 8-bit CPUs and 11-bit offset binary ADCs. The digitization rate (360 samples per second per channel) was chosen to accommodate the use of simple digital notch filters to remove 60 Hz (mains frequency) interference [161, 162].

Various adaptive filter structures similar to shown in Figure 2.3 are developed using NLMS, NSRLMS, NSLMS, NSSLMS, ENLMS, ENSRLMS, ENSLMS and ENSSLMS algorithms. The noise generator detailed in 3.9.1 is used here. In our experiments we have considered a dataset of five ECG records: data100, data105, data108, data203 and data228 to ensure the consistency of results. The simulation results for data 105 are shown in this work. In these experiments we have used first 4000 samples of the ECG signals. Using the dataset all experiments are performed for 10 times and average SNRI values are recorded. The adaptive filter length is chosen as 5, a random noise of variance 0.01 is added to the signals, which resembles the channel noise; the step size μ is taken as 0.01. In our experiments, we have considered four dominant artefacts, namely Power Line Interference (PLI), Baseline Wander (BW), Muscle Artefacts (MA) and Electrode Motion artefacts (EM). To evaluate the performance signal to noise ratio improvement (SNRI) is measured using a MATLAB program based on (3.25), in addition to this MSE, misadjustment, EMSE are also measured using (2.1), (2.2) and (2.4) for ten repeated times and average values are tabulated.

4.7.1. Adaptive Power-line Interference Cancellation

This experiment demonstrates PLI cancellation in ECG signals. The input to the filter is ECG signal corrupted with a PLI of amplitude 1mv, frequency 60Hz and sampled at 200Hz. The reference signal is synthesized sinusoidal noise generated in the noise generator; the output of the filter is recovered signal. The developed ANCs have the same structure shown in Figure 2.3. The contaminated ECG signal is applied as input $x(n) = s_1 + n_1$, the correlated noise reference is applied as n_2 and the output is y(n). Various filter structures are implemented using NLMS, NSRLMS, NSLMS, NSSLMS, ENLMS, ENSRLMS, ENSLMS and ENSSLMS algorithms. The simulation results are shown as follows.

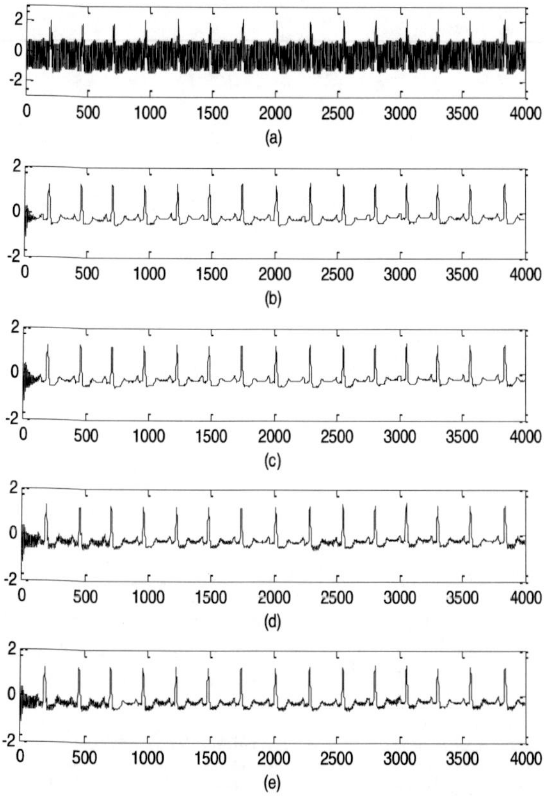

Figure 4.3. Typical filtering results for PLI cancellation using data normalized adaptive filtering techniques: (a) ECG signal with PLI, (b) recovered signal using NLMS algorithm, (c) recovered signal using NSRLMS algorithm, (d) recovered signal using NSLMS algorithm, (e) recovered signal using NSSLMS algorithm.

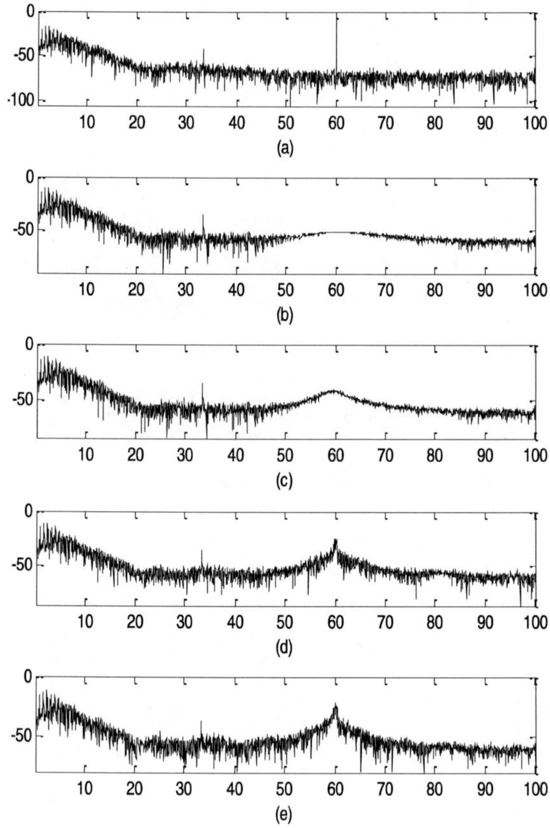

Figure 4.4. Typical frequency spectrums for PLI cancellation using data normalization adaptive filtering techniques: (a) ECG signal with PLI, (b) after NLMS algorithm, (c) after NSRLMS algorithm, (d) after NSLMS algorithm, (e) after NSSLMS algorithm.

Table 4.3. Performance contrast of normalized algorithms for the removal of PLI

Rec. No	NLMS	ENLMS	NSRLMS	NSLMS	NSSLMS	ENSRLMS	ENSLMS	ENSSLMS
100	11.9448	10.9590	11.8964	8.4669	7.3579	9.9511	8.4394	7.2598
105	11.6712	11.4725	11.6284	9.5001	8.4316	10.9466	8.7837	7.9371
108	11.9631	10.2998	11.9131	9.1170	8.3978	9.6220	8.0784	7.2668
203	11.6510	9.8840	11.4207	9.6259	8.4900	9.1281	7.3467	6.5176
228	11.9303	10.4036	12.0163	9.6737	8.0943	8.9463	7.3229	6.9522
Avg.	11.8320	10.4010	11.7749	9.2767	8.1543	9.9204	7.9942	7.1865

From Table 4.3 it is clear that NLMS and ENLMS achieves highest SNRI, but NSRLMS and ENSRLMS achieves SNRI very close to that of NLMS and ENLMS with only single multiplication for the computation of weight update recursion. Whereas NSSLMS and ENSSLMS got SNRI less than their unsigned versions with zero multiplications.

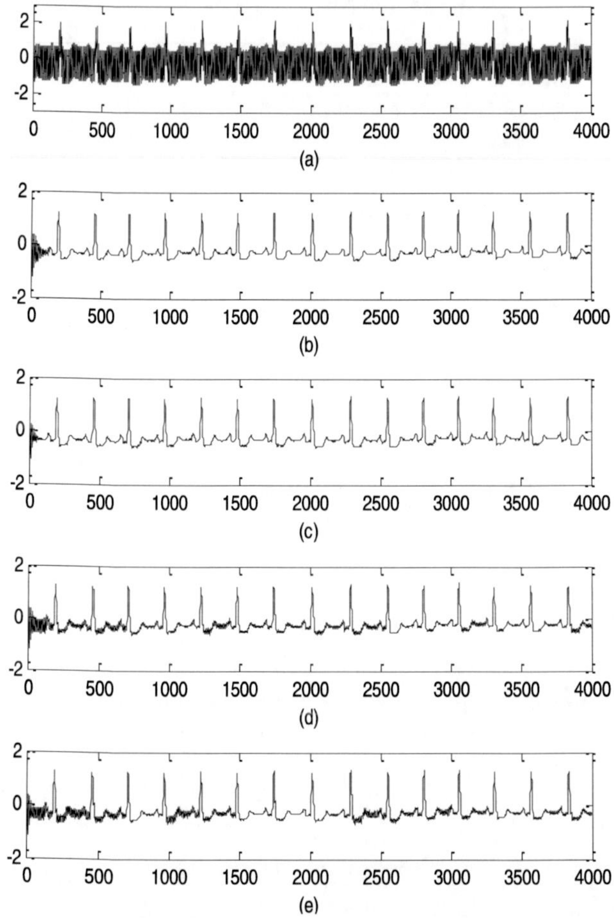

Figure 4.5.Typical filtering results for PLI cancellation using error nonlinear adaptive filtering techniques: (a) ECG signal with PLI, (b) recovered signal using ENLMS algorithm, (c) recovered signal using ENSRLMS algorithm, (d) recovered signal using ENSLMS algorithm, (e) recovered signal using ENSSLMS algorithm.

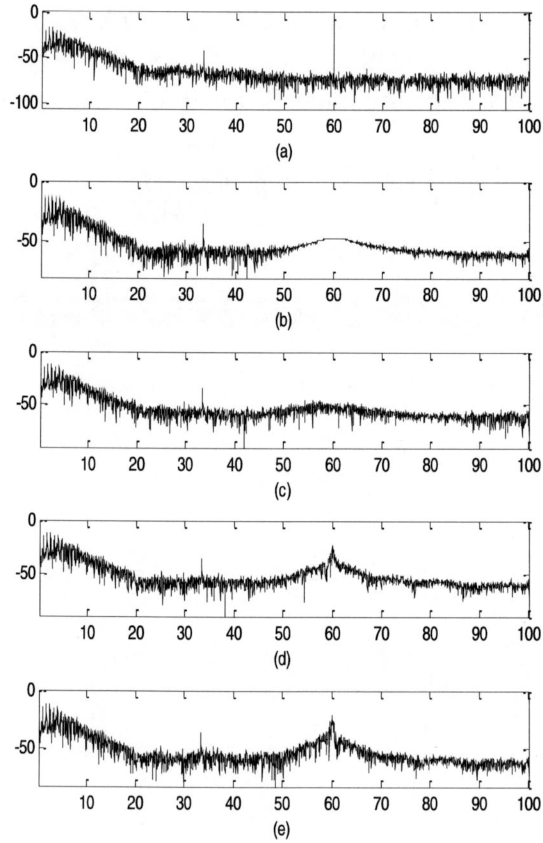

Figure 4.6. Typical frequency spectrums for PLI cancellation using error nonlinear adaptive filtering techniques: (a) ECG signal with PLI, (b) after ENLMS algorithm, (c) after ENSRLMS algorithm, (d) after ENSLMS algorithm, (e) after ENSSLMS algorithm.

Figure 4.7 and 4.8 illustrates the results of the excess mean square error (EMSE) for PLI reduction using data normalized algorithms and error nonlinear algorithms. This phenomenon is also demonstrated in Table 4.7, where the EMSE and M_{ad} for data normalized algorithms are shown. The EMSE and M_{ad} are calculated using (2.4) and (2.2) for different types of artefacts over the data set considered and averaged for ten times. Among the four data normalized algorithms NLMS got minimum EMSE and low M_{ad}, however NSRLMS achieves EMSE and M_{ad} slightly less than that of NLMS with reduced computational complexity.

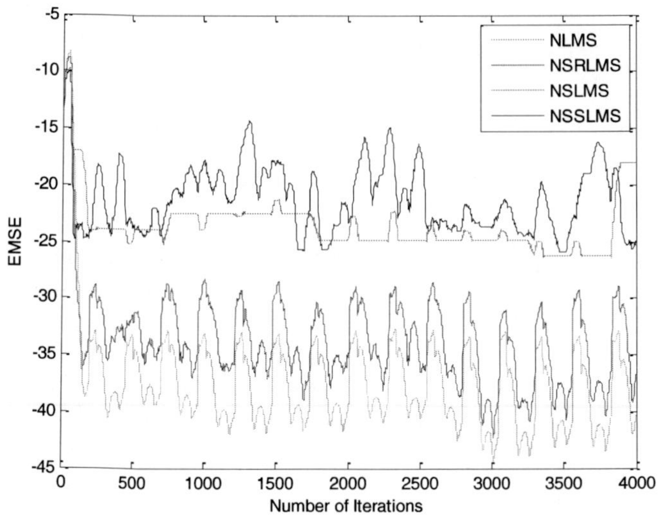

Figure 4.7. EMSE behavior in the PLI cancellation using data normalized adaptive filtering techniques.

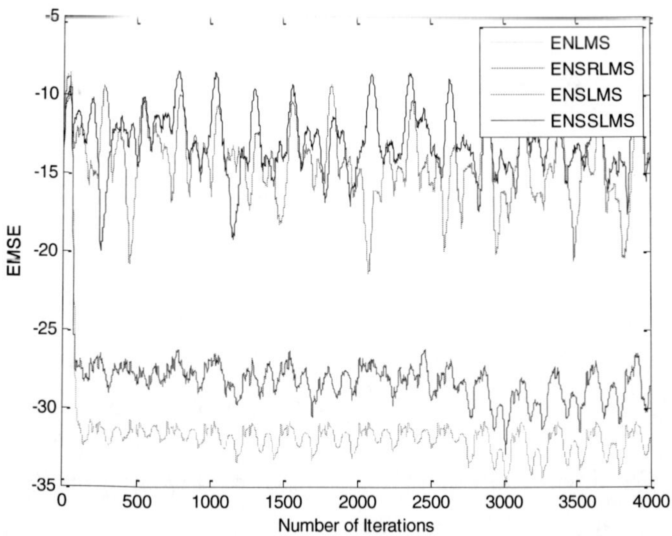

Figure 4.8. EMSE behavior in the PLI cancellation using error nonlinear adaptive filtering techniques.

Similarly, Table 4.8 shows the EMSE and M_{ad} calculations for error nonlinear algorithms, in which ENLMS got less EMSE and M_{ad}, however

ENSRLMS achieves EMSE and M_{ad} slightly less than that of ENLMS with reduced computational complexity.

4.7.2. Adaptive Baseline Wander Removal

This experiment demonstrates BW cancellation, which is a non-stationary noise cancellation. The input to the filter is ECG signal is contaminated with respiration baseline wander; this is applied to a noise canceller shown in Figure 2.3. The reference signal is a real BW obtained from MIT-BIH Noise Stress Test Database. Various filter structures are developed using NLMS, NSRLMS, NSLMS, NSSLMS, ENLMS, ENSRLMS, ENSLMS and ENSSLMS. The simulation results for these ANCs are shown as follows. The SNRI for various filtering methods is calculated using (3.25) and is shown in Table 4.4. The EMSE and M_{ad} are calculated using (2.4) and (2.2) for different types of artefacts over the data set considered and averaged for ten times. A comparison of EMSE and M_{ad} for data normalization is shown in Table 4.7. Figure 4.9 shows the BW removal using data normalized algorithms. Figure 4.10 shows BW removal using error normalized algorithms, Figure 4.11 and Figure 4.12 show EMSE behavior in data normalization and error nonlinear filtering respectively.

Among the four data normalized algorithms NLMS got minimum EMSE and low M_{ad}, however NSRLMS achieves EMSE and M_{ad} slightly less than that of NLMS with reduced computational complexity. Similarly, Table 4.8 shows the EMSE and M_{ad} calculations for error nonlinear algorithms, in which ENLMS got less EMSE and M_{ad}, however ENSRLMS achieves EMSE and M_{ad} slightly less than that of ENLMS with reduced computational complexity.

From Table 4.4 the SNRI for NLMS and ENLMS are better than their signed versions, whereas NSRLMS and ENSRLMS got SNRI slightly less than the NLMS and ENLMS algorithms with reduced number of computations.

Table 4.4. Performance contrast of normalized algorithms for the removal of BW

Rec. No	NLMS	ENLMS	NSRLMS	NSLMS	NSSLMS	ENSRLMS	ENSLMS	ENSSLMS
100	9.0717	8.8932	8.8575	8.2527	6.4445	8.8778	5.9655	5.2152
105	11.6536	10.2891	11.1317	8.8560	7.9423	9.9608	6.8806	5.6840
108	10.0627	9.4489	9.4754	8.7383	6.9345	9.3970	6.9058	6.2174
203	9.1872	8.9971	8.2857	6.7347	5.9609	8.8382	6.4212	5.6292
228	10.8201	8.2755	10.4830	8.9809	7.6581	7.9808	6.8768	5.8804
Avg.	10.1599	9.1807	9.6426	8.3125	6.9880	9.0121	6.6099	5.7252

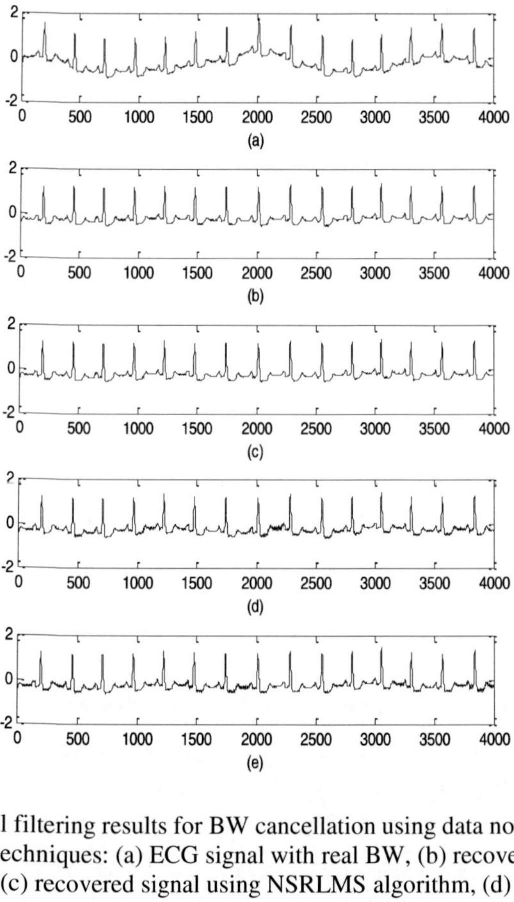

Figure 4.9. Typical filtering results for BW cancellation using data normalization adaptive filtering techniques: (a) ECG signal with real BW, (b) recovered signal using NLMS algorithm, (c) recovered signal using NSRLMS algorithm, (d) recovered signal using NSLMS algorithm, (e) recovered signal using NSSLMS algorithm.

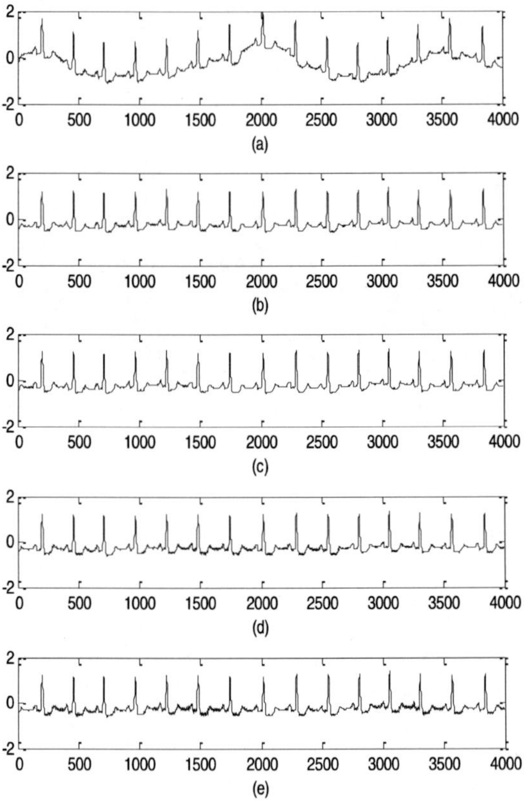

Figure 4.10. Typical filtering results for BW cancellation using error nonlinear adaptive filtering techniques: (a) ECG signal with real BW, (b) recovered signal using ENLMS algorithm, (c) recovered signal using ENSRLMS algorithm, (d) recovered signal using ENSLMS algorithm, (e) recovered signal using ENSSLMS algorithm.

4.7.3. Adaptive Cancellation of Muscle Artefacts

This experiment demonstrates MA cancellation, which is a non-stationary noise cancellation. The input to the filter is ECG signal is contaminated with respiration baseline wander; this is applied to a noise canceller shown in Figure 2.3. The reference signal is a real MA obtained from MIT-BIH Noise Stress Test Database. The MA originally had a sampling frequency of 360Hz and therefore they were anti-alias re-sampled to 128Hz in order to match the sampling rate of the ECG. In the simulated model initially, the weight vector is taken as a null vector. At the initial stage of the filtering the error is maximum, so that the adaptation is slow. As number of feedback loops are going this error decreases because of the adaptation of the weight vector in accordance of the input noisy signal. The process will continue until the error value becomes minimum, i.e., the reference signal becomes closely correlated with the noise component in the ECG signal. Finally, the noise component is getting subtracted due to the trained reference signal because of the adaptive filter. The same analysis can be applied to all the adaptive noise cancellers.

Various filter structures are implemented using NLMS, NSRLMS, NSLMS, NSSLMS, ENLMS, ENSRLMS, ENSLMS and ENSSLMS. The simulation results for these ANCs are shown as follows. The SNRI for various filtering methods is shown in Table 4.5. A comparison of EMSE and M_{ad} is shown in Table 4.7 and Table 4.8. In this case also NLMS, NSRLMS achieves minimum EMSE and M_{ad} respectively. Figure 4.13 shows the MA removal using data normalized algorithms. Figure 4.14 shows MA removal using error nonlinear algorithms. Figure 4.15 and Figure 4.16 show EMSE behavior in data normalization and error nonlinear filtering respectively.

From Table 4.5 the SNRI for NLMS and ENLMS are better than their signed versions, whereas NSRLMS and ENSRLMS got SNRI slightly less than the NLMS and ENLMS algorithms with reduced number of computations.

Table 4.5. Performance contrast of normalized algorithms for the removal of MA

Rec. No.	NLMS	ENLMS	NSRLMS	NSLMS	NSSLMS	ENSRLMS	ENSLMS	ENSSLMS
100	9.2738	8.7608	8.6948	6.6882	5.1890	8.5280	7.2991	6.4621
105	11.1589	10.3248	10.7969	7.8169	6.8141	9.7392	7.9010	6.7238
108	10.2980	9.8435	9.7647	7.6231	5.5868	9.5248	7.6478	6.8086
203	11.9847	9.7120	11.4005	9.6401	8.1926	8.6228	8.1430	7.4127
228	10.1020	9.2147	9.0338	8.069	6.8312	8.8794	7.9096	7.2502
Avg.	10.5634	9.5711	9.9381	7.9674	6.5227	9.0588	7.7801	6.9314

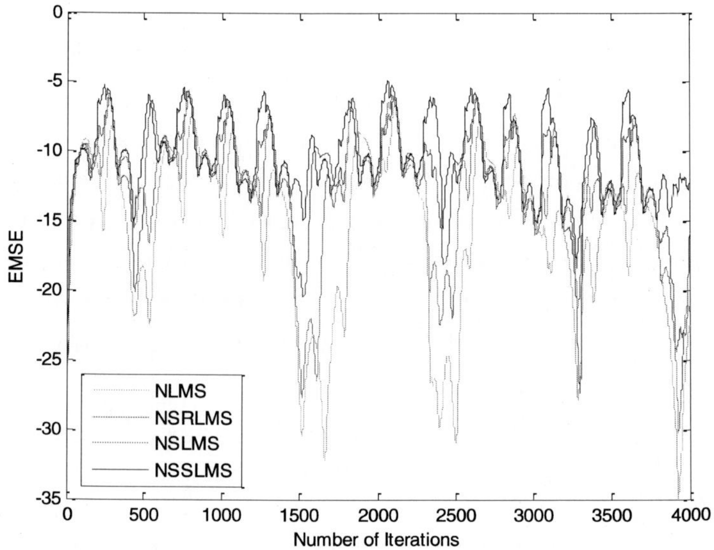

Figure 4.11. EMSE behavior in the BW cancellation using data normalized adaptive filtering techniques.

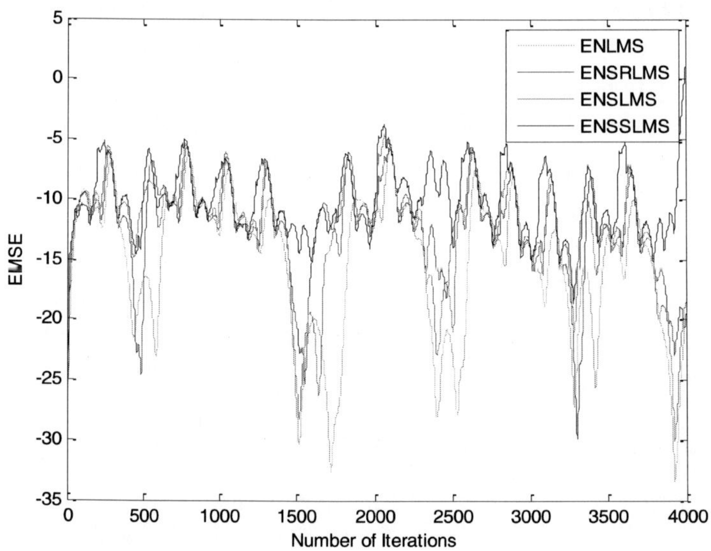

Figure 4.12. EMSE behavior in the BW cancellation using error nonlinear adaptive filtering techniques.

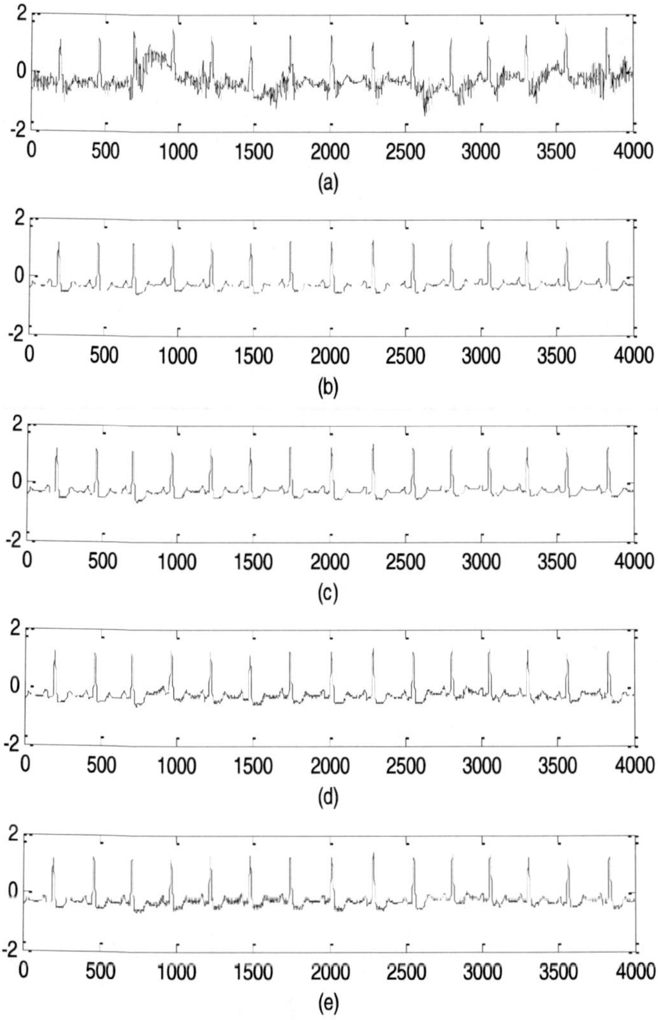

Figure 4.13. Typical filtering results for MA cancellation using data normalization adaptive filtering techniques: (a) ECG signal with real MA, (b) recovered signal using NLMS algorithm, (c) recovered signal using NSRLMS algorithm, (d) recovered signal using NSLMS algorithm, (e) recovered signal using NSSLMS algorithm.

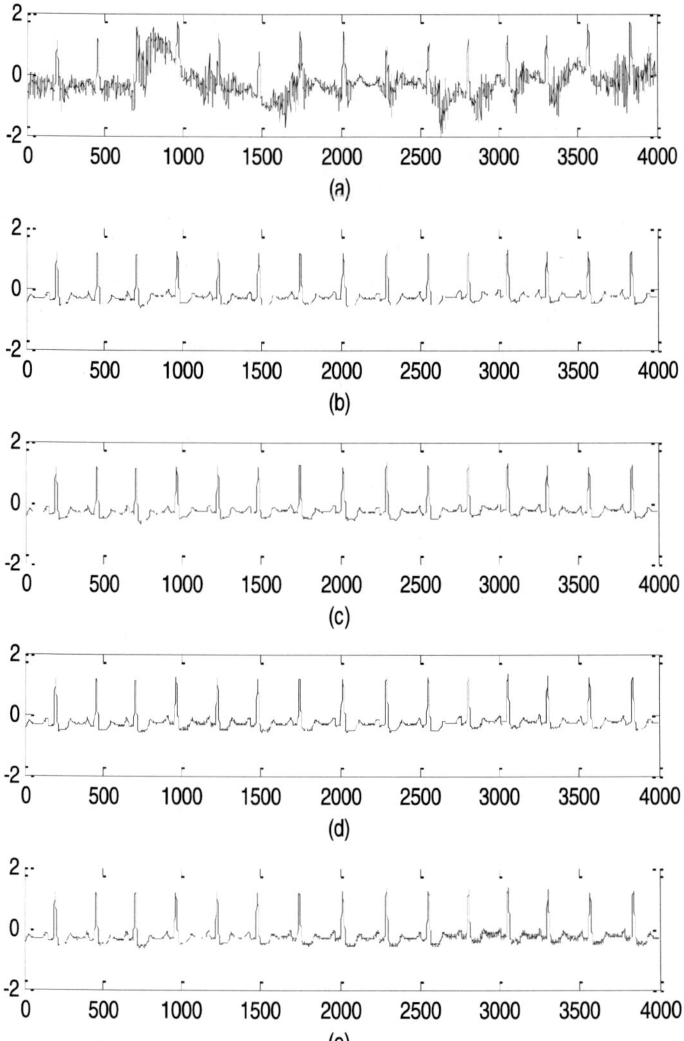

Figure 4.14. Typical filtering results for MA cancellation using error nonlinear adaptive filtering techniques: (a) ECG signal with real MA, (b) recovered signal using ENLMS algorithm, (c) recovered signal using ENSRLMS algorithm, (d) recovered signal using ENSLMS algorithm, (e) recovered signal using ENSSLMS algorithm.

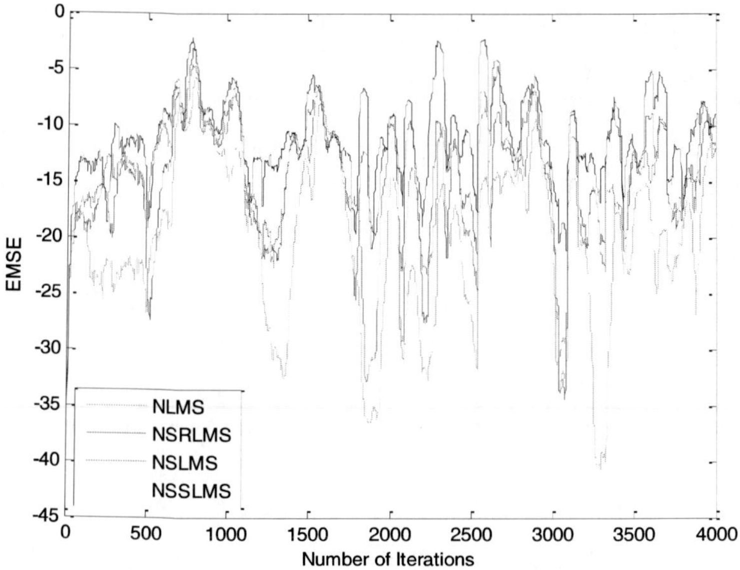

Figure 4.15. EMSE behavior in the MA cancellation using date normalized adaptive filtering techniques.

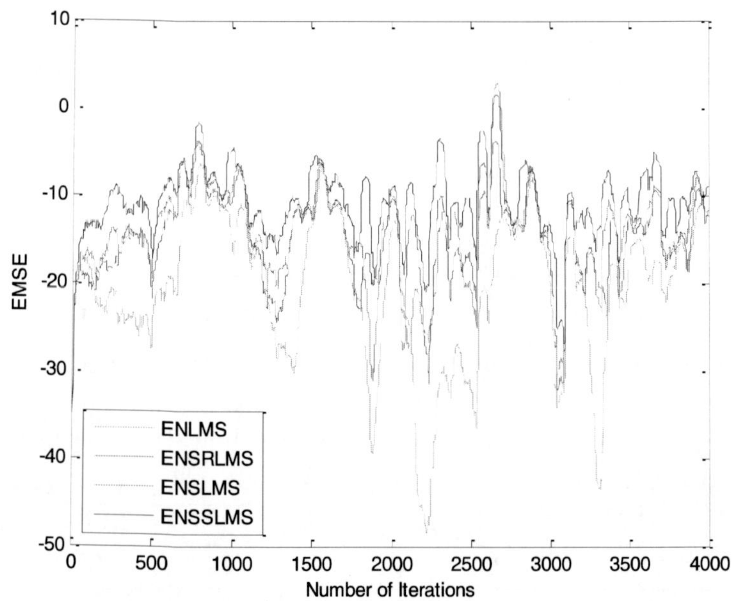

Figure 4.16. EMSE behavior in the MA cancellation using error nonlinear adaptive filtering techniques.

4.7.4. Adaptive Cancellation of Electrode Motion Artefacts

This experiment demonstrates EM cancellation, which is a non-stationary noise cancellation. The input to the filter is ECG signal is contaminated with respiration baseline wander; this is applied to a noise canceller shown in Figure 2.3. The reference signal is a real EM obtained from MIT-BIH Noise Stress Test Database. The EM originally had a sampling frequency of 360Hz and therefore they were anti-alias re-sampled to 128Hz in order to match the sampling rate of the ECG. In the simulated model initially, the weight vector is taken as a null vector. At the initial stage of the filtering the error is maximum. As number of feedback loops are going this error decreases because of the adaptation of the weight vector in accordance of the input noisy signal. The process will continue until the error value becomes minimum, i.e., the reference signal becomes closely correlated with the noise component in the ECG signal. Finally, the noise component is get subtracted due to the trained reference signal because of the adaptive filter. The same analysis can be applied to all the adaptive noise cancellers.

Various filter structures are developed using NLMS, NSRLMS, NSLMS, NSSLMS, ENLMS, ENSRLMS, ENSLMS and ENSSLMS. The SNRI for various filtering methods is calculated using MATLAB program based on (3.25) and shown in Table 4.6. A comparison of EMSE and M_{ad} is shown in Table 4.7 and Table 4.8. Figure 4.17 shows the EM removal using data normalized algorithms. Figure 4.18 shows EM removal using error nonlinear algorithms. Figure 4.19 and Figure 4.20 show EMSE behavior in data normalization and error normalization filtering respectively. In the reduction of electrode motion artefacts both NLMS and ENLMS performs better in terms of SNRI, however NSRLMS and ENSRLMS with single multiplication achieves SNRI slightly less than that of NLMS, ENLMS. Similarly, the EMSE and M_{ad} are slightly inferior to that of NLMS and ENLMS.

Table 4.6. Performance contrast of normalized algorithms for the removal of EM

Rec No.	NLMS	ENLMS	NSRLMS	NSLMS	NSSLMS	ENSRLMS	ENSLMS	ENSSLMS
100	10.9872	10.5729	10.8200	7.8668	7.6165	9.7070	6.8666	6.1584
105	12.8975	10.9500	12.2121	8.9552	8.0493	10.2890	7.5060	6.2268
108	11.1567	9.8545	10.7172	8.6646	6.8205	9.2030	6.8768	5.8618
203	10.2148	9.1975	9.5363	7.9293	7.3478	8.4638	7.0474	6.2606
228	10.5675	9.0285	9.7255	7.9868	7.5365	8.3758	6.8850	5.6010
Avg.	11.1647	9.9206	10.6022	8.2805	7.4741	9.2077	7.0363	6.0217

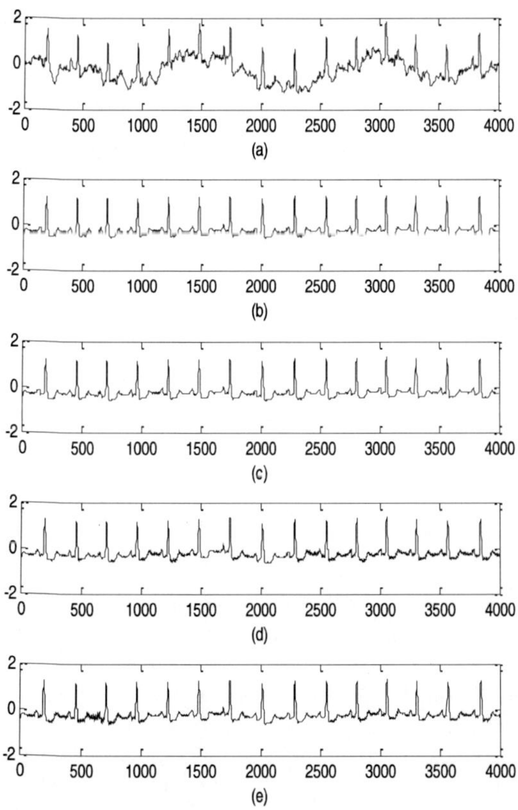

Figure 4.17. Typical filtering results for EM cancellation using data normalization adaptive filtering techniques: (a) ECG signal with real EM, (b) recovered signal using NLMS algorithm, (c) recovered signal using NSRLMS algorithm, (d) recovered signal using NSLMS algorithm, (e) recovered signal using NSSLMS algorithm.

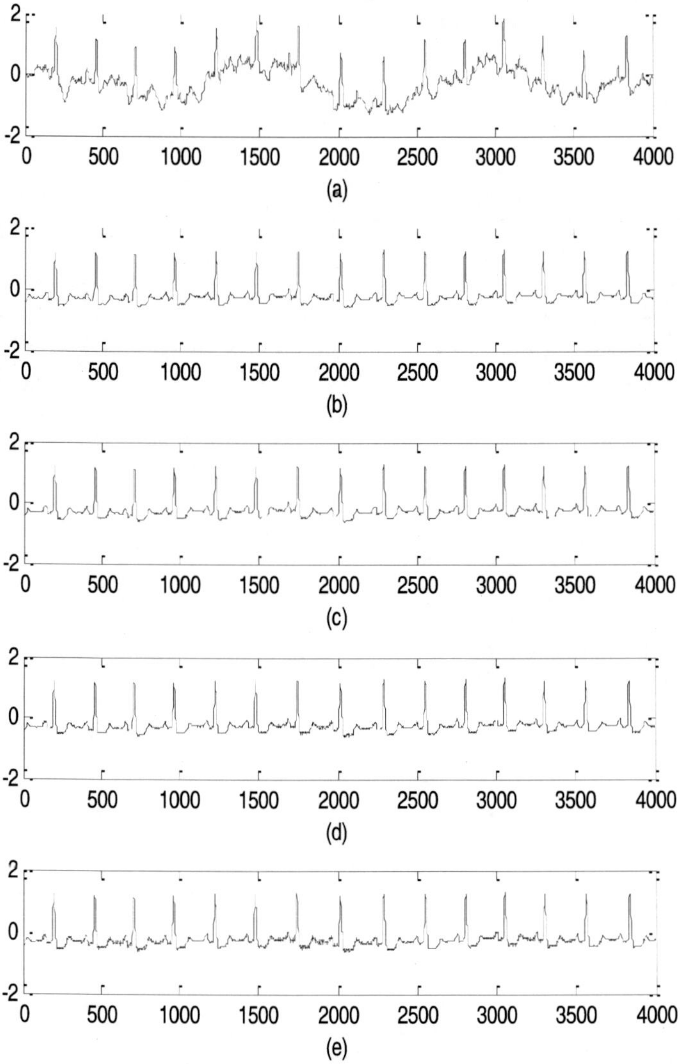

Figure 4.18. Typical filtering results for EM cancellation using error nonlinear adaptive filtering techniques: (a) ECG signal with real EM, (b) recovered signal using ENLMS algorithm, (c) recovered signal using ENSRLMS algorithm, (d) recovered signal using ENSLMS algorithm, (e) recovered signal using ENSSLMS algorithm.

Table 4.7. A comparison of EMSE and M_{ad} for various artifacts using data normalized algorithms

Noise Type	Record Number	NLMS		NSRLMS		NSLMS		NSSLMS	
		EMSE	M_{ad}	EMSE	M_{ad}	EMSE	M_{ad}	EMSE	M_{ad}
PLI	100	-35.4423	0.0022	-32.9680	0.0038	-20.5313	0.0673	-18.0426	0.1193
	105	-38.1297	0.0021	-36.5779	0.0038	-23.2150	0.0328	-20.4403	0.0621
	108	-35.6593	0.0022	-33.3122	0.0038	-22.1957	0.0495	-20.3312	0.0760
	203	-33.3277	0.0018	-30.2508	0.0036	-23.2823	0.0181	-20.5606	0.0339
	228	-36.1993	0.0024	-34.0340	0.0040	-23.6570	0.0436	-19.6323	0.1102
	Average	**-35.7478**	**0.0021**	**-33.4285**	**0.0038**	**-22.5763**	**0.0422**	**-19.8014**	**0.0803**
BW	100	-11.4784	0.5409	-10.1241	0.7388	-10.0132	0.7579	-9.4152	0.8698
	105	-14.8997	0.3527	-12.2614	0.5144	-11.4546	0.6194	-9.3859	0.7922
	108	-11.5508	0.5741	-10.2390	0.7766	-10.1252	0.7972	-9.5217	0.9161
	203	-10.8257	0.3185	-9.4676	0.4354	-8.3142	0.5679	-7.0235	0.7644
	228	-12.9327	0.5152	-11.3445	0.7427	-11.1337	0.7796	-10.3252	0.9392
	Average	**-12.3374**	**0.4602**	**-10.6873**	**0.6415**	**-10.2081**	**0.7044**	**-9.1343**	**0.8563**
MA	100	-14.2363	0.2866	-11.7764	0.5050	-11.2207	0.5739	-8.3371	101148
	105	-15.6156	0.1887	-12.1586	0.4184	-11.8929	0.4448	-9.3836	0.7926
	108	-14.0474	0.3231	-12.0121	0.5163	-11.1570	0.6286	-9.2472	0.9758
	203	-13.7262	0.1633	-11.3159	0.2845	-10.2308	0.3652	-8.0495	0.6036
	228	-16.1641	0.2448	-13.2561	0.4782	-12.7259	0.5403	-9.9798	1.0169
	Average	**-14.7579**	**0.2413**	**-12.1038**	**0.4404**	**-9.4454**	**0.5105**	**-8.9994**	**0.9007**
EM	100	-12.0061	0.4790	-10.4112	0.6915	-10.3107	0.7077	-9.5258	0.8479
	105	-13.5054	0.3068	-11.8758	0.4465	-10.5551	0.6052	-9.2236	0.8224
	108	-12.1006	0.5059	-10.8103	0.6809	-10.2360	0.7771	-9.4003	0.9420
	203	-10.8006	0.3203	-9.5932	0.4230	-8.1075	0.5955	-6.5766	0.8472
	228	-13.7872	0.4232	-12.2511	0.6028	-11.6622	0.6903	-10.3049	0.9436
	Average	**-12.4399**	**0.4070**	**-10.9883**	**0.5689**	**-10.1743**	**0.6751**	**-9.0062**	**0.8806**

Table 4.8. A comparison of EMSE and M_{ad} for various artifacts using error nonlinear algorithms

Noise Type	Record Number	ENLMS		ENSRLMS		ENSLMS		ENSSLMS	
		EMSE	M_{ad}	EMSE	M_{ad}	EMSE	M_{ad}	EMSE	M_{ad}
PLI	100	-31.1493	0.0058	-28.6078	0.0132	-18.9691	0.0837	-17.3116	0.1064
	105	-31.7629	0.0046	-29.2064	0.0104	-19.8722	0.0920	-17.5291	0.1142
	108	-31.8542	0.0054	-29.4589	0.0117	-19.4843	0.0978	-17.5610	0.1250
	203	-31.7581	0.0026	-29.2588	0.0058	-20.1058	0.0797	-17.5498	0.0991
	228	-32.1326	0.0062	-29.6635	0.0138	-19.4612	0.0962	-17.4066	0.0816
	Average	**-31.7314**	**0.0049**	**-29.2390**	**0.0109**	**-19.5785**	**0.0898**	**-17.4716**	**0.1052**
BW	100	-11.3451	0.5577	-10.0901	0.7446	-9.8778	0.7819	-7.5092	0.9490
	105	-12.5583	0.3816	-10.9719	0.5498	-10.7962	0.5725	-9.0546	0.8550
	108	-11.8461	0.5364	-10.2013	0.7834	-10.2507	0.7745	-3.3048	0.9337
	203	-10.6737	0.3298	-9.4175	0.4405	-9.0982	0.4741	-7.3138	0.7150
	228	-12.8608	0.5238	-11.0913	0.7873	-11.2885	0.7523	-7.1966	0.8502
	Average	**-11.8568**	**0.4658**	**-10.3544**	**0.6611**	**-10.2622**	**0.6710**	**-6.8758**	**0.8605**
MA	100	-13.9836	0.3038	-11.1686	0.5808	-11.3217	0.5607	-8.7457	0.6259
	105	-15.4987	0.1939	-12.1481	0.4194	-10.7437	0.5795	-8.8212	0.9022
	108	-14.4282	0.2960	-11.2392	0.6168	-12.4234	0.4696	-5.8529	0.8321
	203	-14.5691	0.1345	-11.4592	0.2753	-11.7774	0.2558	-8.1069	0.5956
	228	-16.2474	0.2402	-12.0209	0.6356	-13.4664	0.6556	-4.9206	0.9599
	Average	**-14.9454**	**0.2340**	**-11.6072**	**0.4655**	**-11.9465**	**0.5042**	**-7.2894**	**0.7831**
EM	100	-11.9244	0.4881	-10.2533	0.7171	-10.1015	0.7426	-8.5079	0.8718
	105	-13.4472	0.3110	-11.3067	0.4090	-11.6878	0.5663	-8.2076	0.9391
	108	-12.6225	0.4486	-10.5162	0.7286	-10.9138	0.6648	-8.9973	0.8336
	203	-11.2157	0.2911	-9.3247	0.4500	-9.1756	0.4857	-7.4776	0.7409
	228	-13.7395	0.4279	-11.8788	0.6567	-11.4923	0.7178	-9.5700	0.9075
	Average	**-12.5898**	**0.3933**	**-10.6559**	**0.5922**	**-10.6742**	**0.6354**	**-8.5520**	**0.8585**

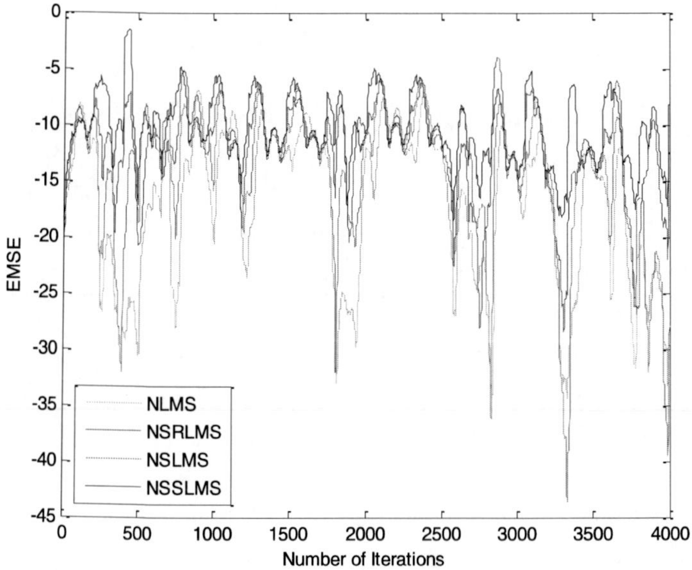

Figure 4.19. EMSE behavior in the EM cancellation using data normalized adaptive filtering techniques.

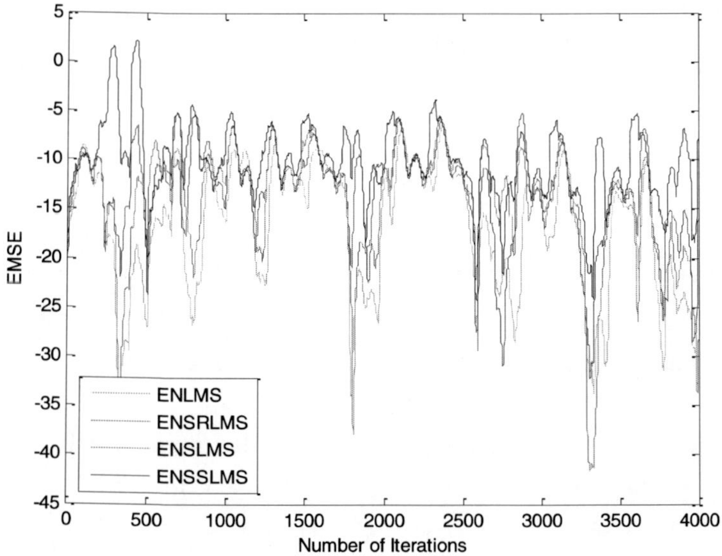

Figure 4.20. EMSE behavior in the EM cancellation using error nonlinear adaptive filtering techniques.

4.8. CONCLUSION

In this chapter the problem of noise cancelation from ECG signal using sign based normalized adaptive filters are developed and tested on real signals with different artefacts obtained from the MIT-BIH database by developing adaptive noise cancellers using MATLAB as shown in the Figure 2.3. For this, the input and the desired response signals are properly chosen in such a way that the filter output is the best least squared estimate of the original ECG signal. Here we have considered two types of normalized filters i.e., data normalized and error normalized. These are commonly known as NLMS and ENLMS algorithms respectively. In order to reduce computational complexity, we have successfully developed various ANCs using sign-based versions of both NLMS and ENLMS. Between NLMS and ENLMS the performance of NLMS is found to be better in terms of SNRI, EMSE and M_{ad}. From the two normalized version algorithms we obtain six sign-based versions of algorithms, totally six sign based and two normalized ANCs are developed for ECG denoising. Among six sign-based algorithms NSRLMS got first place, next goes to ENSRLMS and then NSLMS, NSSLMS, ENSLMS, ENSSLMS in the descending order. The filtering performance of all the eight algorithms is better than LMS algorithm, whereas the computational complexity is less than that of LMS except one division operation is needed for normalization. From the simulation results based on SNRI, EMSE and misadjustment calculations it is clear that the proposed sign-based ANCs remove non-stationary noise efficiently. The proposed treatment provides high signal to noise ratio with less computational complexity. Hence the sign based normalized algorithms are more suitable in wireless biotelemetry ECG systems. Among all the algorithms we have chosen NSRLMS and ENSRLMS based ANCs for development in real time environment on embedded digital signal processor.

Chapter 5

BLOCK BASED ADAPTIVE FILTERING TECHNIQUES FOR THE REMOVAL OF NOISE IN ECG SIGNALS

5.1. INTRODUCTION TO BLOCK ADAPTIVE FILTERS

In real time biotelemetry applications, the signal length is quite large i.e., a large number of samples are processed; it may require adaptive filters with excessively long lengths. In such cases the conventional LMS algorithm, which is simple, is computationally complex to implement. The block processing of the data samples can significantly reduce the computational complexity of adaptive filters. In block implementation, a block of samples of the filter input and desired output are collected and then processed together to obtain a block of output samples. Thus, the processing involves serial to parallel conversion of the input data, parallel processing of the collected data and parallel to serial conversion of the generated output data. The computational burden of the adaptive filter can then be reduced significantly through elegant parallel processing of the data samples. Thus, a good measure of the computational complexity in a block processing system is given by the number of operations required to process one block of data divided by the block length. The sharing of the processing time among the samples in each block is the key to achieve high computational efficiency. To minimize computational complexity and improve filtering capability of the noise cancellers we have implemented various adaptive noise cancellers based on block processing of data samples to remove artefacts from ECG signals, presented below. The summary of algorithms used in this chapter is given in Table 5.1.

Table 5.1. Summary of algorithms used in Chapter 5

S. No	Acronym	Name	Advantage
1.	BLMS	Block least mean square	It processes signal by portioned in to non-overlapping blocks in time domain
2.	FBLMS	Fast block least mean square	It processes signal by portioned in to non-overlapping blocks in frequency domain
3.	BNLMS	Block normalized least mean square	It processes signal by portioned in to non-overlapping blocks in time domain with fast convergence
4.	FBNLMS	Fast block normalized least mean square	It processes signal by portioned in to non-overlapping blocks in frequency domain with fast convergence
5.	BENLMS	Block error nonlinear least mean square	It processes signal by portioned in to non-overlapping blocks in time domain with fast convergence
6.	FBENLMS	Fast block error nonlinear least mean square	It processes signal by portioned in to non-overlapping blocks in frequency domain with fast convergence
7.	BBNLMS	Block based normalized least mean square	Fast convergence, avoids gradient noise amplification problem, process the signal with overlapping blocks
8.	BBNSRLMS	Block based normalized sign regressor least mean square	Fast convergence, avoids gradient noise amplification problem, only one multiplication needed to compute the recursion, process the signal with overlapping blocks
9.	BBNSLMS	Block based normalized sign least mean square	Fast convergence, avoids gradient noise amplification problem, it requires L MACs, process the signal with overlapping blocks
10.	BBNSSLMS	Block based normalized sign sign least mean square	Fast convergence, avoids gradient noise amplification problem, zero multiplications required, enter recursion is computed with addition with sign check operation, process the signal with overlapping blocks

S. No	Acronym	Name	Advantage
11.	BBENLMS	Block based error nonlinear least mean square	Fast convergence, minimizes signal distortion, process the signal with overlapping blocks
12.	BBENSRLMS	Block based error nonlinear sign regressor least mean square	Fast convergence, minimizes signal distortion, only one multiplication needed to compute the recursion
13.	BBENSLMS	Block based error nonlinear sign least mean square	Fast convergence, minimizes signal distortion, it requires L MACs, process the signal with overlapping blocks
14.	BBENSSLMS	Block based error nonlinear sign sign least mean square	Fast convergence, minimizes signal distortion, zero multiplications required, enter recursion is computed with addition with sign check operation, process the signal with overlapping blocks

5.1.1. The Block LMS (BLMS) Algorithm

Consider a BLMS based adaptive filter, depicted in Figure 5.1, that takes an input sequence $\boldsymbol{x}(n)$, which is partitioned into non-overlapping blocks of length P each by means of a serial-to-parallel converter, and the blocks of the data so produced are applied to an FIR filter of length L, one block at a time. The tap weights of the filter are updated after the collection of each block of data samples, so that the adaptation of the filter proceeds on a block-by-block basis rather than on a sample-by-sample basis as in conventional LMS algorithm [100].

The filter coefficients are updated from block to block as,

$$\boldsymbol{w}(j+1) = \boldsymbol{w}(j) + \mu \sum_{i=0}^{P-1} \boldsymbol{x}(jP+i)e(jP+i) \qquad (5.1)$$

k refers to the block index.

$\boldsymbol{w}(j) = [w_0\,(j), w_1(j), \dots, w_{P-1}(j)]^t$is the tap weight vector corresponding to the j-th block, $\boldsymbol{x}(jP+i) = [x(jP+i), x(jP+i-1), \dots, x(jP+i-P+1)]^t$ and $e(jP+i)$ is the output error given by,

$$e(jP + i) = d(jP + i) - y(jP + i) \tag{5.2}$$

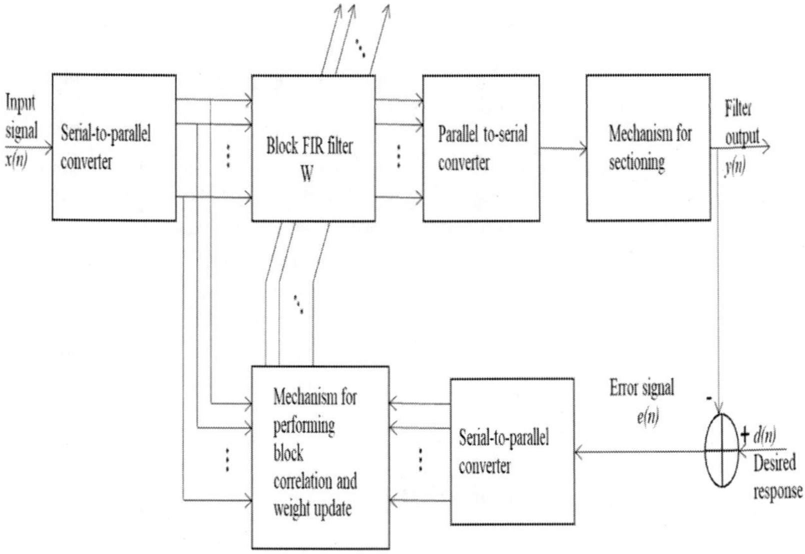

Figure 5.1. Block adaptive filter.

Since, in the block LMS algorithm, the error signal is allowed to vary at the sampling rate, it follows that, for each block of data, we have different values of the error signal for use in the adaptive process. Accordingly, for the jth block, we sum the product $\boldsymbol{x}(jP+i)e(jP+i)$ over all possible values of "i" for the formation of weight recursion equation given by (5.1).

The sequence $d(jP + i)$ is so-called desired response available during the initial training period and $y(jP + i)$ is the filter output given as,

$$y(jP + i) = \boldsymbol{w}^{\boldsymbol{t}}(j)\boldsymbol{x}(jP + i) \tag{5.3}$$

The parameter μ popularly called the step size parameter is to be chosen as $0 < \mu < \frac{2}{P*tr\,R}$ for convergence of the algorithm.

The BLMS has the same properties as those of the conventional LMS algorithm. The fundamental difference between them lies in the estimates of the gradient vector used in their respective implementations. The BLMS uses a more accurate estimate of the gradient vector because of the time averaging, with the estimation accuracy increasing as the block size P is increased. With reference to block length P and filter length L, in BLMS the following are three possible choices, each with its own practical implications:

1. P = L, this is an optimal choice from the viewpoint of computational complexity.
2. P < L, this offers an advantage of reduced processing delay. Moreover, this results an adaptive filter computationally efficient than the LMS algorithm.
3. P > L, gives rise to redundant operations in the adaptive process, because the estimation of the gradient vector uses more information than the filter itself.

In our experiments we have developed the optimal choice i.e., P = L.

5.1.2. Frequency Domain Implementation of BLMS Algorithm

The computational burden of the block LMS algorithm lies between, a linear convolution of the tap inputs and tap weights of the filter, a linear correlation between the tap inputs of the filter and the error signal. The fast Fourier transform (FFT) algorithm provides a powerful tool for performing fast convolution and fast correlation. The fast block LMS (FBLMS) algorithm is nothing but a fast implementation of the BLMS algorithm in frequency domain. In FBLMS the filter parameters are adapted in the frequency domain by using FFT algorithm. The element by element multiplication of the frequency domain samples of the input and filter coefficients is followed by an IFFT and a proper windowing of the result to obtain the output vector [86]. Linear convolution of time domain sequences can be efficiently implemented using frequency domain processing. Here the signals are transformed from time domain to frequency domain and backwards using the FFT and IFFT, respectively. From signal processing theory, we know that the overlap save method and overlap add method provides two efficient procedures for fast convolution, i.e., computation of linear convolution using discrete Fourier transform. The overlap save method is the more common one of the two for filtering techniques. As a result, frequency domain implementation of BLMS algorithm is widely used to improve computational efficiency and convergence rate due to the use of FFT [102] – [106].

The filter output vector as given by (5.3) is obtained by convolving the input data sequence **x**(n) with the filter coefficient vector $w_0(j), w_1(j), \ldots, w_{L-1}(j)$ and thus can be realized efficiently by the overlap-save method via $M = L + P - 1$ point FFT, where the first $L - 1$ points come from the previous sub-block, for which the output is to be discarded. Similarly, the weight update term in (5.1), viz., $\sum_{r=0}^{P-1} \boldsymbol{x}(jP + r)e(jP + r)$ can be obtained by the usual circular correlation technique, by employing M point FFT and setting the last $P - 1$ output terms as zero [71]. This technique can be used for the efficient implementation FBLMS algorithm. In this algorithm an N-point FFT is used for the computation, where $N = 2M$. Thus, the N-by-1 vector is given by,

$$\boldsymbol{W}(j) = FFT\begin{bmatrix}\boldsymbol{w}(j)\\ 0\end{bmatrix} \tag{5.4}$$

denote the FFT coefficients of the zero padded, tap weight vector **w** (j). In the above equation 0 is the *M-by*-1 null vector. The frequency domain weight vector **W** (j) is twice as long as the time domain weight vector **w** (j). Let **X** (j) is diagonal matrix obtained by Fourier transforming two successive blocks of input data,

$$\mathbf{X}(k) = diag\{FFT[u(kL - L), \ldots, u(kL - 1), u(kL), \ldots, u(kL + L - 1)]\} \tag{5.5}$$

and **d** (*j*) is the L-by-1 desired response vector.

By applying overlap-save method to the linear convolution of (5.3) yields the L-by-1 vector,

$$\boldsymbol{Y}^T(k) = \text{last L elements of IFFT } [\mathbf{X}(j)\,\mathbf{W}(j)]. \quad (5.6)$$

Now the corresponding L-by-1 error signal vector is given by

$$\boldsymbol{e}(j) = \boldsymbol{d}(j) - \boldsymbol{y}(j) \quad (5.7)$$

In the implementation of linear convolution described in (5.6), the first L elements are discarded from the output.

The error signal vector **e** (j) in frequency domain is represented as,

$$\boldsymbol{E}(j) = FFT\begin{bmatrix}\mathbf{0}\\ \boldsymbol{e}(j)\end{bmatrix} \quad (5.8)$$

Finally, the weight update recursion in (5.1) can be realized in frequency domain as,

$$\boldsymbol{W}(j+1) = \boldsymbol{W}(j) + \mu FFT\begin{bmatrix}\boldsymbol{\Phi}(j)\\ \mathbf{0}\end{bmatrix} \quad (5.9)$$

Therefore in FBLMS, the filtering and weight updating will be done in frequency domain using FFT i.e., convolution is efficiently done by block processing further by applying FFT for the entire block. Here $\boldsymbol{\Phi}$ (j) is a matrix of first M elements of IFFT [**D** (j) **X** (j) **E** (j)]. Where **D** (j) is related to diagonal matrix of average signal power, **X** (j) is diagonal matrix obtained by Fourier transforming two successive blocks of input data, **E** (j) is transform of error signal vector.

Figure 5.2 depicts a flow graph of the FBLMS algorithm, which shows the realization of filtering, error estimation and tap-weight adaptation. The input samples are collected in an input buffer whose output is the vector **x**(j), consisting of L new samples and $N-1$ sample from the previous block. The vector **x**(j) is converted to the frequency domain and multiplied by the associated tap-weight vector, on element by element basis. This gives the samples of the filter output in the frequency domain which is subsequently converted to the time domain using an IFFT.

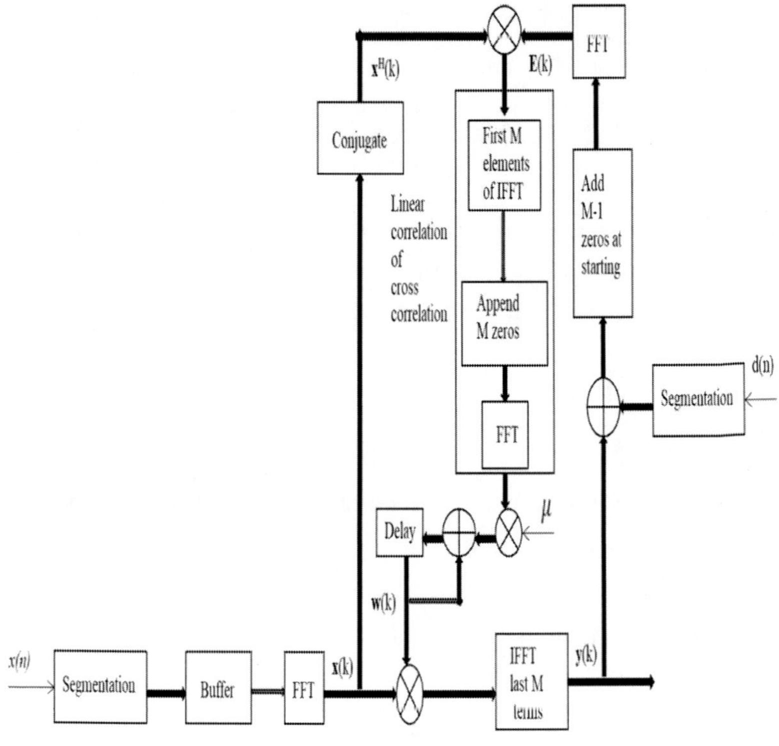

Figure 5.2. Schematic flow graph of the FBLMS algorithm.

5.1.3. The Block Normalized LMS (BNLMS) Algorithm

The BLMS algorithm allows the filter coefficients to be adjusted once per output block increasing the processing speed. However, both LMS and BLMS suffer from the drawback of gradient noise amplification and low convergence speed. The so called normalized LMS algorithm overcomes both these two drawbacks by considering the variation in the signal level at the filter output and selecting the normalized step size parameter that results in a stable as well as fast converging algorithm. Therefore, the convergence behavior of the BLMS algorithm is greatly improved if we replace the scalar step-size parameter μ by a diagonal matrix μ(*n*) in (5.1) whose diagonal elements are the set of normalized step-size parameters.

The variable step size μ(*n*) is given by (4.2), for convenience it is given below.

$$\mu(n) = \frac{\mu}{\varepsilon + ||\boldsymbol{x}(n)||2}$$

The parameter ε is set to avoid denominator being too small and step size parameter too big, μ(*n*) is nonlinear variable of input signal, which changes along with ε. The step diminishes and accelerates convergence process.

Comparing (2.17) and (4.4), the update equation of NLMS is a scaled version of LMS algorithm. Therefore, the convergence behavior of the BLMS algorithm is greatly improved if we replace the scalar step-size parameter μ by a diagonal matrix μ(*n*) in (5.1) whose diagonal elements are the set of normalized step-size parameters. The resultant update equation corresponds to block normalized LMS algorithm. The weight update equation is given as,

$$\boldsymbol{w}(j+1) = \boldsymbol{w}(j) + \mu(n) \sum_{r=0}^{P-1} \boldsymbol{x}(jP+r) e(jP+r) \tag{5.10}$$

The size of the change to weight vector **w**(n) is therefore be in inversely proportional to the norm of data vector **x**(n). The data vector **x**(n) with a large norm will generally lead to a small change to **w**(n) than a vector with a smaller norm. This normalization results smaller step size values than conventional LMS. The normalized algorithm usually converges faster than the LMS algorithm, since it utilizes a variable convergence factor aiming at the minimization of the instantaneous output error.

5.1.4. The Block Error Nonlinear LMS (BENLMS) Algorithm

The advantage of ENLMS algorithm is that the step size can be chosen independent of the input signal power and the number of tap weights. Hence the ENLMS algorithm has a convergence rate and a steady state error better than LMS algorithm. The combination of ENLMS and BLMS results BENLMS. The update equation of BENLMS is similar to (5.1) expect μ is replaced with $\beta(n)$ given in (4.7), for convenience it is given below.

$$\beta(n) = \frac{\mu}{\varepsilon + \|e(n)\|^2}$$

Now the weight update recursion for BENLMS can be written as,

$$w(j+1) = w(j) + \beta(n) \sum_{r=0}^{P-1} u(jP+r)e(jP+r) \tag{5.11}$$

A common major drawback of adaptive noise cancellers using LMS-based algorithms is the large value of excess mean-square error which results in signal distortion in the noise-canceled signal. In BENLMS algorithm the time-varying step-size is inversely proportional to squared norm of error vector rather than input data vector as in BNLMS algorithm.

5.1.5. Frequency Domain Implementation of BNLMS and BENLMS Algorithms

The realization of BNLMS and BENLMS algorithms follows the same methodology as that of for FBLMS. The frequency domain versions of BNLMS and BENLMS are known as fast BNLMS (FBNLMS) and fast BENLMS (FBENLMS) algorithms. By using (5.9), (4.2) and (4.7) the weight update recursions for FBNLMS and FBENLMS are written as follows.

$$\boldsymbol{W}(j+1) = \boldsymbol{W}(j) + \mu(n)FFT\begin{bmatrix}\boldsymbol{\Phi}(j)\\ 0\end{bmatrix} \tag{5.12}$$

and

$$\boldsymbol{W}(j+1) = \boldsymbol{W}(j) + \beta(n)FFT\begin{bmatrix}\boldsymbol{\Phi}(j)\\ \mathbf{0}\end{bmatrix} \tag{5.13}$$

Where $\mu(n)$ and $\beta(n)$ are variable step sizes due to data and error normalizations respectively.

In biotelemetry applications the physiological, non-physiological and channel noises mask the features of the ECG signal. Moreover, in practical cases large data rates are used to send the bulk data in less time. In order to process such bulk data, the conventional filter length has to be increased, the computational complexity of the filter increases. In this aspect to reduce the complexity FFT based block processing is the suitable candidate.

5.2. Extension to Block Processing of NLMS Based Adaptive Filters

To reduce the computational complexity, we adopt block processing of normalized algorithms discussed in Chapter 4. But at this time, we consider overlapping blocks. Unlike BLMS algorithm, here we take single error value for calculating the output. The additional computations required to compute the variable step size for all the algorithms discussed in Chapter 4 can be further reduced by using this block-based approach in which the input data is partitioned into blocks and the maximum magnitude within each block is used to compute variable step size parameter.

With this, the weight update relations for NLMS as given by (4.4) and its sign based versions NSRLMS, NSLMS and NSSLMS given by (4.8)-

(4.10) takes the following form. Now the weight update relation of Block Based NLMS (BBNLMS) algorithm for $x_{Li} \neq 0$ and $\varepsilon = 0$ is written as,

$$\boldsymbol{w}(n+1) = \boldsymbol{w}(n) + \frac{\mu}{x_{Li}^2}\boldsymbol{x}(n)e(n) \tag{5.14}$$

Similarly, the weight update relations for Block Based NSRLMS (BBNSRLMS), Block Based NSLMS (BBNSLMS) and Block Based NSSLMS (BBNSSLMS) algorithms are written as follows,

$$\boldsymbol{w}(n+1) = \boldsymbol{w}(n) + \frac{\mu}{x_{Li}^2} Sign\{\boldsymbol{x}(n)\}\, e(n); \tag{5.15}$$

$$\boldsymbol{w}(n+1) = \boldsymbol{w}(n) + \frac{\mu}{x_{Li}^2}\boldsymbol{x}(n) Sign\{e(n)\}; \tag{5.16}$$

and

$$\boldsymbol{w}(n+1) = \boldsymbol{w}(n) + \frac{\mu}{x_{Li}^2} Sign\{\boldsymbol{x}(n)\} Sign\{e(n)\}; \tag{5.17}$$

where, $x_{Li} = \max\{|x_k|, k \in Z_i'\}, Z_i' = \{iL, iL+1, \ldots, iL+L-1\}, i \in Z$, and for $x_{Li} = 0$ and $\varepsilon = 0$ the equations (5.14)-(5.17) becomes $\mathbf{w}(n+1) = \mathbf{w}(n)$.

5.3. Extension to Block Processing of ENLMS Based Adaptive Filters

Similar to BBNLMS and its signed versions, we have implemented the block-based algorithms for ENLMS algorithm and its signed versions. Due to block processing the ENLMS algorithm with recursion given by (4.5) and its signed based versions ENSRLMS, ENSLMS and ENSSLMS given by (4.11) – (4.13) takes the following form.

Now the weight update relation of Block Based ENLMS (BBENLMS) algorithm for $e_{Li} \neq 0$ and $\varepsilon = 0$ is written as,

$$\boldsymbol{w}(n+1) = \boldsymbol{w}(n) + \frac{\mu}{e_{Li}^2}\boldsymbol{x}(n)e(n) \tag{5.18}$$

Similarly, the weight update relations for Block Based ENSRLMS (BBENSRLMS), Block Based ENSLMS (BBENSLMS) and Block Based ENSSLMS (BBENSSLMS) algorithms are written as follows,

$$\boldsymbol{w}(n+1) = \boldsymbol{w}(n) + \frac{\mu}{e_{Li}^2} Sign\{\boldsymbol{x}(n)\}\, e(n); \tag{5.19}$$

$$\boldsymbol{w}(n+1) = \boldsymbol{w}(n) + \frac{\mu}{e_{Li}^2}\boldsymbol{x}(n) Sign\{e(n)\}; \tag{5.20}$$

and

$$\boldsymbol{w}(n+1) = \boldsymbol{w}(n) + \frac{\mu}{e_{Li}^2} Sign\{\boldsymbol{x}(n)\} Sign\{e(n)\}; \tag{5.21}$$

where,$e_{Li} = \max\{|e_k|, k \in Z_i'\}, Z_i' = \{iL, iL+1, \dots, iL+L-1\}, i \in Z$, and for $x_{Li} = 0$ and $\varepsilon = 0$ the equations (5.18)-(5.21) becomes $\mathbf{w}(n + 1) = \mathbf{w}(n)$.

5.4. Computational Complexity Issues

In FBLMS the major computational block is an *M*- point FFT/IFFT. the FBLMS algorithm consists of two M-point complex multiplications (one for obtaining the filter output in frequency domain, the other for evaluating the weight update term $\mathbf{X}^H(k)$ $\mathbf{E}(k)$ in frequency domain), two *M*-point real multiplications to compute μ $\mathbf{X}^H(k)$ $\mathbf{E}(k)$ and one M-point complex addition for updating the weight vector in frequency domain. Moreover, *P* floating point FP real additions are required to compute error. Noting that the FBLMS algorithm contains a total of 5 *M*-point FFT/IFFT, each FFT/IFFT contains $\log_2^M$ (= *r; say*) stages, each stage consists *M* 2 butterflies, a total of $10Mr+10M$ MAC, $35Mr+18M+2P$ shift, $15Mr + 6M + P$ EC, $30Mr + 22M + P$ EA and $10Mr + 2M + P$ FxP additions are required in the FP based realization. Table 5.2 shows the computational complexity of Block LMS algorithm and its variants.

As the sign-based algorithms are largely free from the MAC operations, the proposed schemes provide elegant means to remove noise from the ECG signal. Table 5.3 shows the computational complexity of various overlapping block based normalized signed algorithms.

Table 5.2. Computational complexity comparison of BLMS and its variants in time domain and frequency domain ($M = L + P - 1, r = \log_2^{M}$)

Algorithm	MAC	ASC	Divisions	Shift
BLMS	$(L+1)P+L$	Nil	Nil	$(L+P)$
FBLMS	$10Mr+10M$	$10Mr+2M+P$	Nil	$35Mr+18M+2P$
BNLMS	$(L+1)P+2L$	Nil	L	$(L+P)$
FBNLMS	$10Mr+10M+L$	$10Mr+2M+P$	L	$35Mr+18M+2P$
BENLMS	$(L+1)P+2L$	Nil	L	$(L+P)$
FBENLMS	$10Mr+10M+L$	$10Mr+2M+P$	L	$35Mr+18M+2P$

Table 5.3. Computational complexity comparison of block based normalized signed algorithms

Algorithm	MACs	ASC	Divisions
BBNLMS	L+2	Nil	1
BBNSRLMS	1	Nil	1
BBNSLMS	L	Nil	1
BBNSSLMS	Nil	L	1
BBENLMS	L+2	Nil	1
BBENSRLMS	1	Nil	1
BBENSLMS	L	Nil	1
BBENSSLMS	Nil	L	1

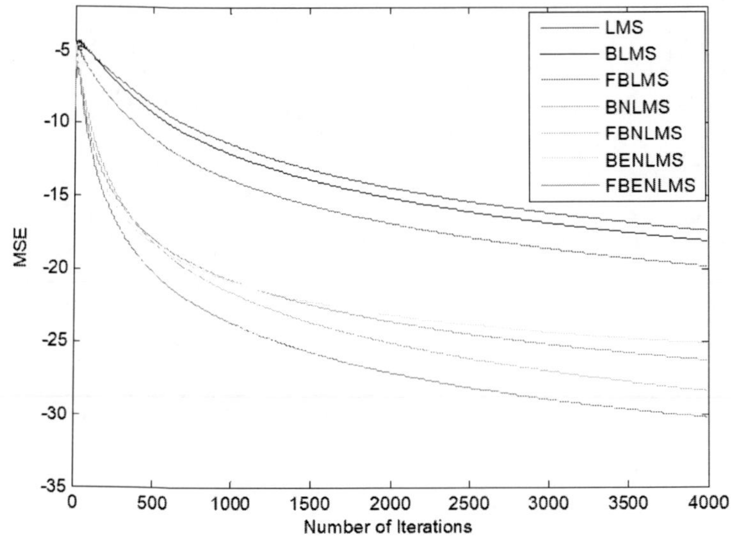

Figure 5.3. Convergence curves of BLMS and its variants in time domain and frequency domain.

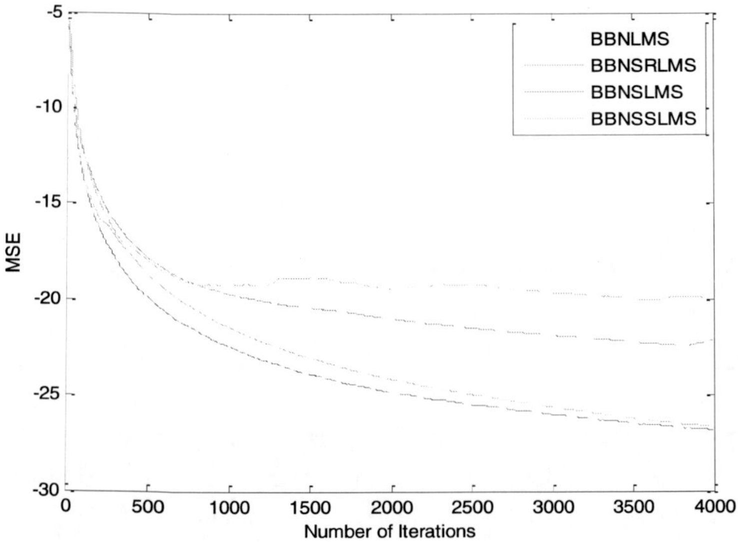

Figure 5.4. Convergence curves of BBNLMS algorithm and its sign-based algorithms.

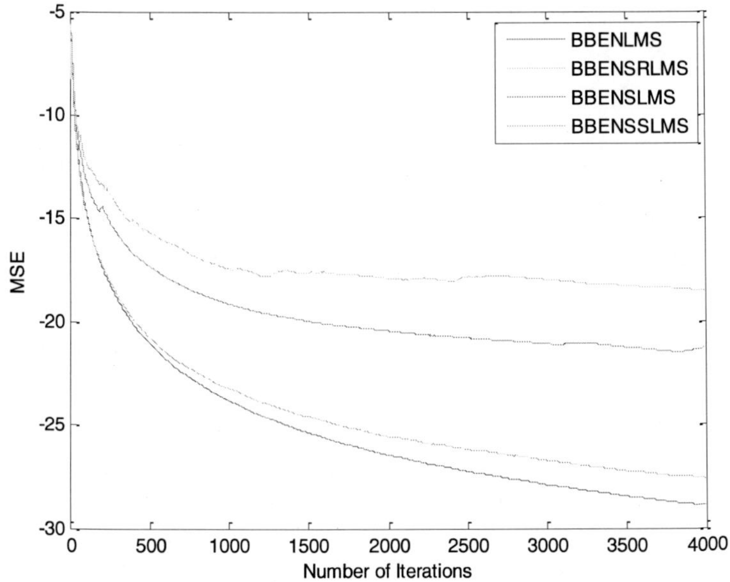

Figure 5.5. Convergence curves of BBENLMS algorithm and its sign-based algorithms.

5.5. Convergence Analysis

The convergence curves of BLMS and its variants in both time domain and frequency domain are shown in Figure 5.3. From the figure it is clear that the convergence characteristics of BLMS are approximately similar to that of LMS algorithm. However, by adopting normalization fast convergence is achieved in both BNLMS and BENLMS algorithms. Because of normalization, the step size varies iteratively; this step size is proportional to the inverse of the total expected energy of the instantaneous values of the coefficients of the input data vector. The BNLMS and BENLMS algorithms usually converge faster than the LMS algorithm, since it utilizes a variable convergence factor aiming at the minimization of the instantaneous output error. The advantage of the BNLMS and BENLMS algorithms is that the step size can be chosen independent of the input signal power and the number of tap weights. Hence these algorithms has a convergence rate and a steady state error better than BLMS algorithm. As a result of frequency domain implementation, the FBLMS algorithm is widely used to improves the convergence rate due to the use of FFT.

The convergence curves of Block based normalized signed algorithms are shown in Figure 5.4 and Figure 5.5. Here block processing improves the convergence characteristics but in its signed versions, because of the presence of signum convergence rate becomes slow moreover some tiny residual noise remains along the ST segment of the ECG signal. The parameters MSE, M_{ad} and EMSE are measured using MATLAB programs based on the (2.1), (2.2) and (2.4) for convergence characterization.

5.6. RESULTS AND DISCUSSIONS

To test the ability of the BLMS, its variants in both time domain and frequency domain, block based normalized algorithms, its variants discussed in this chapter we performed various experiments on real ECG signals with a wide variety of wave morphologies. The BLMS, its variants and block based normalized algorithms; its variants are two different independent categories of block adaptive filters. However, we have considered both categories in noise removal experiments and compared individually. In the former case we process non-overlapping blocks, where as in the latter case we process overlapping blocks.

We used the benchmark MIT-BIH arrhythmia database ECG [110] records as the reference to our work. The MIT-BIH Arrhythmia Database contains 48 half-hour excerpts of two-channel ambulatory ECG recordings, obtained from 47 subjects studied by the BIH Arrhythmia Laboratory ages 23 years to 89 years. Twenty-three recordings were chosen at random from a set of 4000 24-hour ambulatory ECG recordings collected from a mixed population of inpatients (about 60%) and outpatients (about 40%) at Boston's Beth Israel Hospital; the remaining 25 recordings were selected from the same set to include less common but clinically significant arrhythmias that would not be well-represented in a small random sample.

The recordings were digitized at 360 samples per second per channel with 11-bit resolution over a 10 mV range. About half (25 of 48 complete records, and reference annotation files for all 48 records) of this database has been freely available online since PhysioNet's inception in September 1999. The 23 remaining signal files were also available on PhysioNet since February 2005.

The ECG recordings were made using Del Mar Avionics model 445 two-channel reel-to-reel Holter recorders, and the analog signals were recreated for digitization using a Del Mar Avionics model 660 playback unit. The computers used for digitization were designed and built in our laboratory, including the tape-drive controllers and the analog-to-digital converter (ADC) inter-faces; they used then state-of-the-art 1 MHz 8-bit CPUs and 11-bit offset binary ADCs. The digitization rate (360 samples per second per channel) was chosen to accommodate the use of simple digital notch filters to remove 60 Hz (mains frequency) interference [161]-[162].

In our experiments we have considered a dataset of five ECG records: data100, data105, data108, data203 and data228 to ensure the consistency of results, the simulation results for data 105 are shown. We have used 4000 samples of these signals for our experiments. Using these records, we performed our experiments for 10 times and average SNRI is tabulated. We have developed and tested BLMS based adaptive filters in which both the filter length and block length is equal, which is the optimum case. Various adaptive filter structures similar to shown in Figure 2.3 are implemented using BLMS, BNLMS, BENLMS, FBLMS, FBNLMS and FBENLMS. In addition to this we have performed experiments using various ANCs based on BBNLMS, BBNSRLMS, BBNSLMS, BBNSSLMS, BBENLMS, BBENSRLMS, BBENSLMS and BBENSSLMS algorithms. The noise generator detailed in 3.9.1 is used here. For evaluating the performance of the proposed filter structures, we have measured the signal-to-noise ratio improvement (SNRI) in decibels (dBs) using MATLAB program based on the following relation and compared with conventional LMS algorithm.

$$SNRI[db] = SNR_{output} - SNR_{input} = 10log\left(\frac{\sum_i |x_d(n) - x(n)|^2}{\sum_i |x_n(n) - x(n)|^2}\right)$$

where x denotes the clean ECG, x_d is the denoised signal and x_n represents the noisy ECG signal. Similar to SNRI, the parameters MSE, M_{ad} and EMSE are measured using MATLAB programs based on the (2.1), (2.2) and (2.4). In our experiments, we have considered four dominant artefacts, namely Power Line Interference (PLI), Baseline Wander (BW), Muscle Artefacts (MA) and Electrode Motion artefacts (EM). To evaluate the performance signal to noise ratio improvement (SNRI) is measured.

5.6.1. Adaptive Power-Line Interference Cancellation

This experiment demonstrates PLI cancellation in ECG signals. The input to the filter is ECG signal corrupted with a PLI of amplitude 1mv, frequency 60Hz and sampled at 200Hz. The reference signal is synthesized sinusoidal noise generated in the noise generator; the output of the filter is recovered signal. The developed ANCs have the same structure shown in Figure 2.3. The contaminated ECG signal is applied as input $x(n) = s_1 + n_1$, the correlated noise reference is applied as n_2 and the output is y(n). Various filter structures are implemented using non-overlapping block filters BLMS, BNLMS, BENLMS, FBLMS, FBNLMS, FBENLMS and overlapping block filters BBNLMS, BBNSRLMS, BBNSLMS, BBNSSLMS, BBENLMS, BBENSRLMS, BBENSLMS and BBENSSLMS algorithms. The simulation results for adaptive PLI removal using BLMS, its variants are shown in Figure 5.6 and Figure 5.7. The corresponding frequency spectrums of ECG signal at the output of various ANCs are shown in Figure 5.8 and Figure 5.9. The SNRI contrast for this case is shown in Table 5.3. Figure 5.10 illustrates the results of the excess mean square error (EMSE) for PLI reduction using BLMS and its variants in time, frequency domains. This phenomenon is also demonstrated in Table 5.11 and Table 5.12. The EMSE and M_{ad} are calculated for different types of artefacts over the data set considered and average values are taken.

From the figure it is observed that the amplitude of the ECG signals is attenuated. This is because of the signal averaging. The BLMS uses a more accurate estimate of the gradient vector because of the time averaging, with the estimation accuracy increasing as the block size P is increased. The filtering capability of BLMS based ANC is better than that of LMS, moreover the smoothing capability of BLMS algorithm is better. This is demonstrated in Figure 5.8. However due to attenuation the SNRI of this filter is less. From Table 5.4 it is clear that frequency domain filtering greatly increases signal resolution in terms of SNRI, among the three frequency domain filters FBENLMS based ANC filters PLI efficiently.

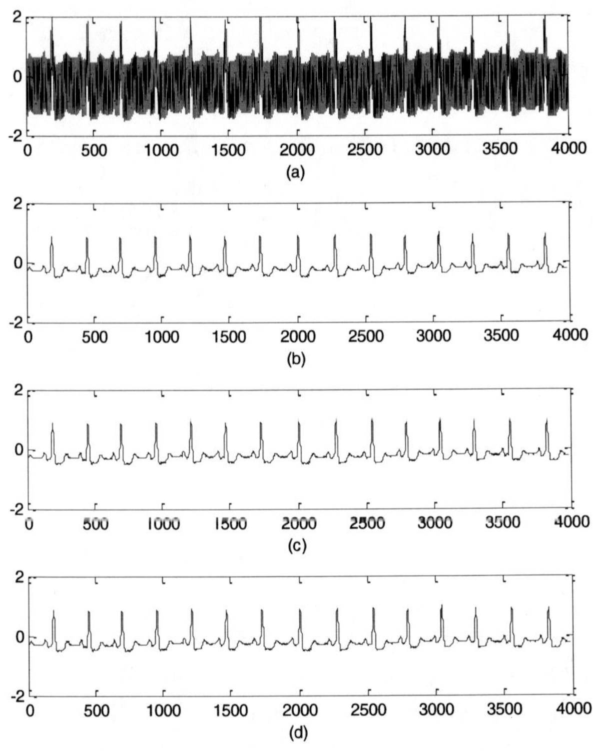

Figure 5.6. Typical filtering results for PLI cancellation using BLMS and its variants in time domain: (a) ECG signal with PLI, (b) recovered signal using BLMS algorithm, (c) recovered signal using BNLMS algorithm, (d) recovered signal using BENLMS algorithm.

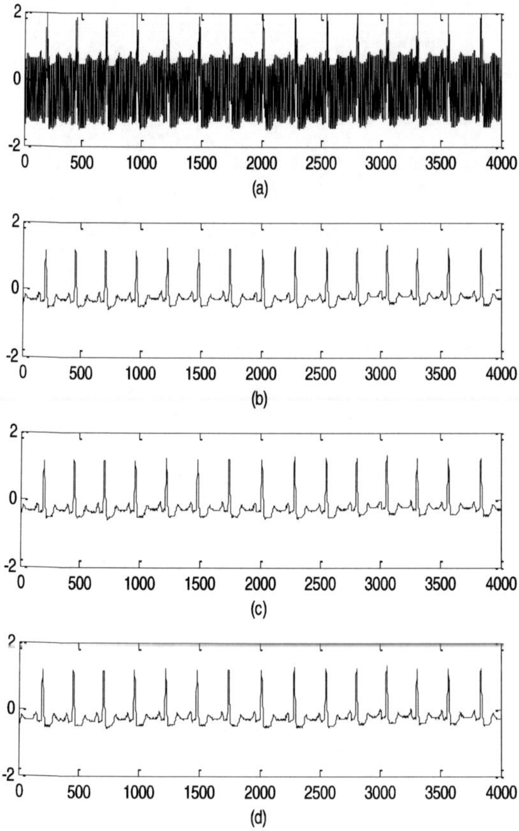

Figure 5.7. Typical filtering results for PLI cancellation using FBLMS and its variants in frequency domain: (a) ECG signal with PLI, (b) recovered signal using FBLMS algorithm, (c) recovered signal using FBNLMS algorithm, (d) recovered signal using FBENLMS algorithm.

Table 5.4. Performance contrast of block adaptive filters for the removal of PLI

Rec. No.	BLMS	FBLMS	BNLMS	FBNLMS	BENLMS	FBENLMS
100	8.3182	21.3666	9.0236	22.3960	10.4213	24.9941
105	8.0068	18.2938	9.9876	19.3076	11.1556	21.3048
108	8.9214	19.7332	9.4105	21.8205	11.7789	23.4052
203	7.9946	17.9358	8.6860	18.1707	9.5700	21.1139
228	7.8338	18.8847	8.7843	20.1583	9.8765	22.0877
Average	8.2149	19.2428	9.0584	20.3706	10.5604	22.5811

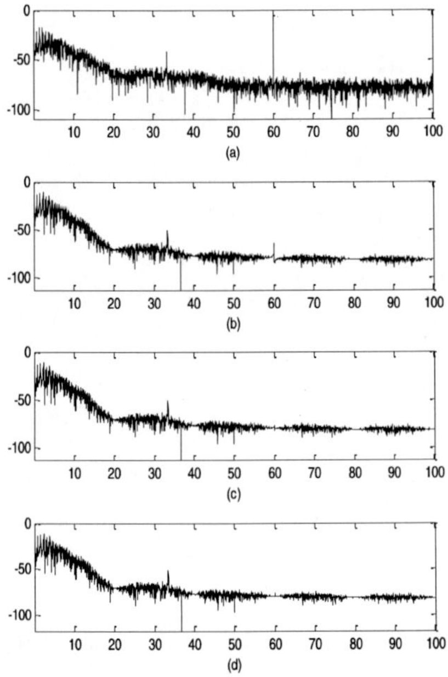

Figure 5.8. Typical frequency spectrums for PLI cancellation using BLMS and its variants in time domain: (a) ECG signal with PLI, (b) recovered signal using BLMS algorithm, (c) recovered signal using BNLMS algorithm, (d) recovered signal using BENLMS algorithm.

From the frequency spectrum shown above it is clear that the proposed ANCs removing the power line interference component efficiently.

The simulation results for adaptive PLI removal using block based normalized algorithms and its signed versions are shown in Figure 5.11 and Figure 5.12. The corresponding frequency spectrums of ECG signal at the output of various ANCs are shown in Figure 5.13 and Figure 5.14. The SNRI contrast for this case is shown in Table 5.5.

Figure 5.15 and Figure 5.16 illustrate the results of the EMSE for PLI reduction using BBNLMS, BBENLMS and its sign-based versions. This phenomenon is also demonstrated in Table 5.14 and Table 5.15. The EMSE and M_{ad} are calculated for different types of artefacts over the data set considered and average values are taken.

From Table 5.5 it is clear that BBENSRLMS performs better than others in signed based block algorithms, next place goes to BBNSRLMS.

Table 5.5. Performance contrast of Block based normalized adaptive filters for the removal of PLI

Rec. No.	BBNLMS	BBENLMS	BBNSRLMS	BBNSLMS	BBNSSLMS	BBENSRLMS	BBENSLMS	BBENSSLMS
100	12.2530	12.9958	11.6596	8.4834	7.7717	12.6976	9.8134	8.3247
105	11.7812	13.4091	10.7868	8.7158	8.3982	12.9371	9.6323	9.1273
108	12.2972	11.9785	9.7595	8.0130	7.8503	11.5313	9.2009	8.9058
203	11.9784	10.8190	9.5021	7.9741	7.0428	10.3276	8.6192	7.2985
228	11.9871	10.7931	9.3588	7.5293	7.9374	10.0717	8.6027	7.7477
Average	12.0613	11.9991	10.2133	8.1431	8.8000	11.5130	9.1737	8.2808

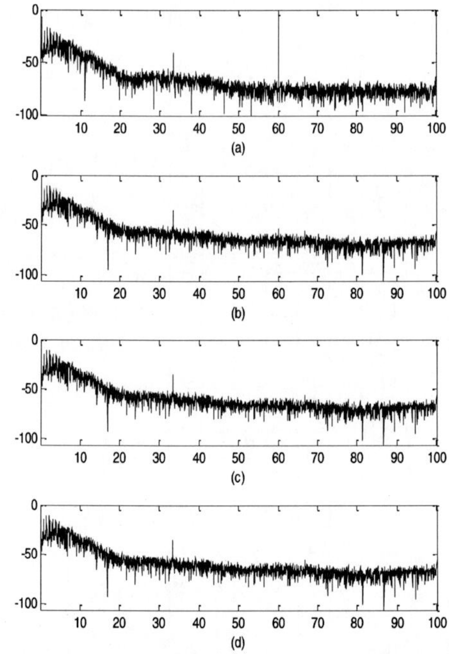

Figure 5.9. Typical frequency spectrums for PLI cancellation using FBLMS and its variants in frequency domain: (a) ECG signal with PLI, (b) recovered signal using FBLMS algorithm, (c) recovered signal using FBNLMS algorithm, (d) recovered signal using FBENLMS algorithm.

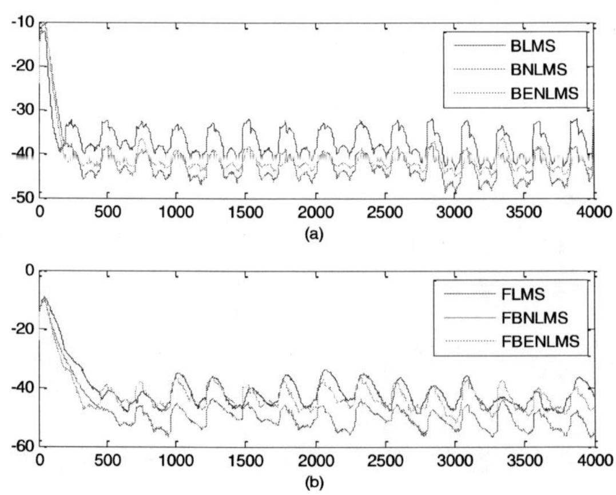

Figure 5.10. EMSE behavior in the PLI cancellation using block adaptive filtering techniques.

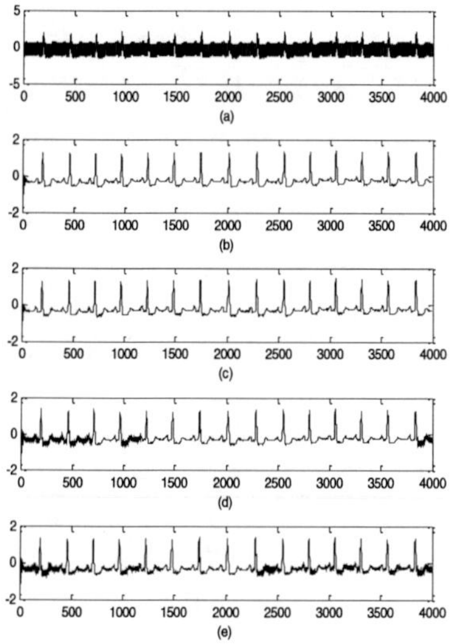

Figure 5.11. Typical filtering results for PLI cancellation using block based data normalized adaptive filtering techniques: (a) ECG signal with PLI, (b) recovered signal using BBNLMS algorithm, (c) recovered signal using BBNSRLMS algorithm, (d) recovered signal using BBNSLMS algorithm, (e) recovered signal using BBNSSLMS algorithm.

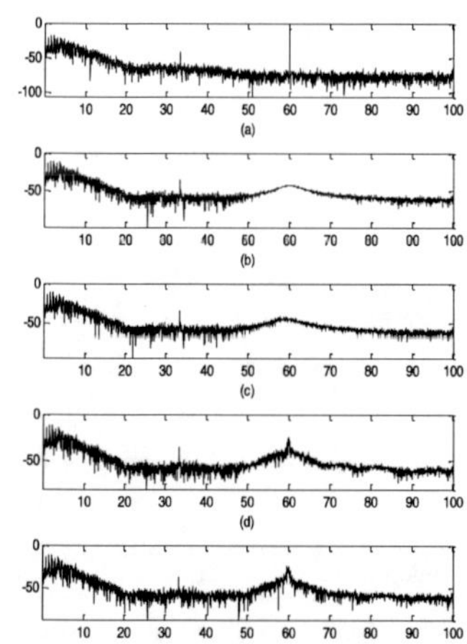

Figure 5.12. Typical frequency spectrums for PLI cancellation using block based data normalized adaptive filtering techniques: (a) ECG signal with PLI, (b) recovered signal using BBNLMS algorithm, (c) recovered signal using BBNSRLMS algorithm, (d) recovered signal using BBNSLMS algorithm, (e) recovered signal using BBNSSLMS algorithm.

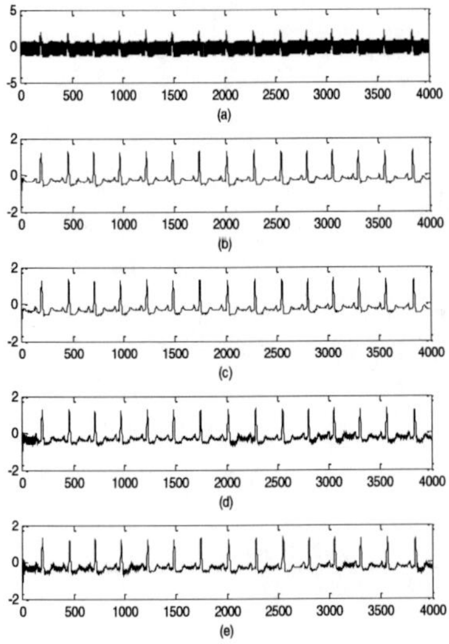

Figure 5.13. Typical filtering results for PLI cancellation using block based error nonlinear adaptive filtering techniques: (a) ECG signal with PLI, (b) recovered signal using BBENLMS algorithm, (c) recovered signal using BBENSRLMS algorithm, (d) recovered signal using BBENSLMS algorithm, (e) recovered signal using BBENSSLMS algorithm.

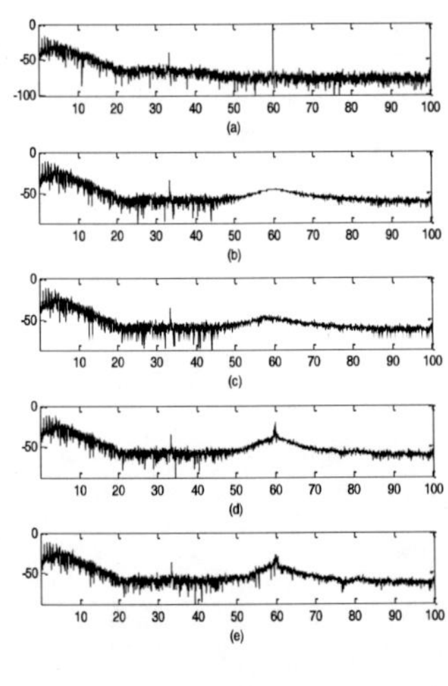

Figure 5.14. Typical frequency spectrums for PLI cancellation using block based error nonlinear adaptive filtering techniques: (a) ECG signal with PLI, (b) recovered signal using BBENLMS algorithm, (c) recovered signal using BBENSRLMS algorithm, (d) recovered signal using BBENSLMS algorithm, (e) recovered signal using BBENSSLMS algorithm.

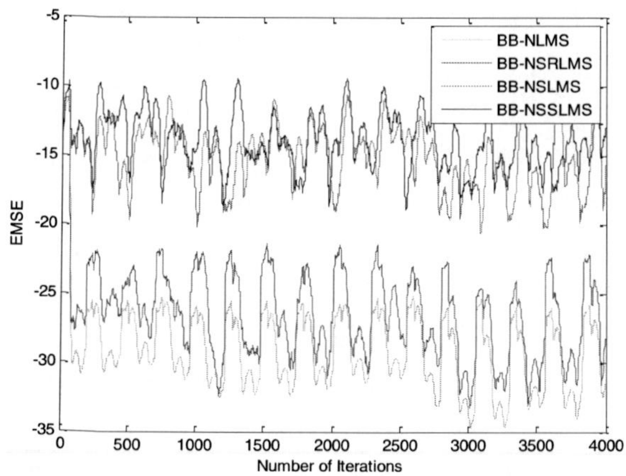

Figure 5.15. EMSE behavior in the PLI cancellation using block-based data normalized adaptive filtering techniques.

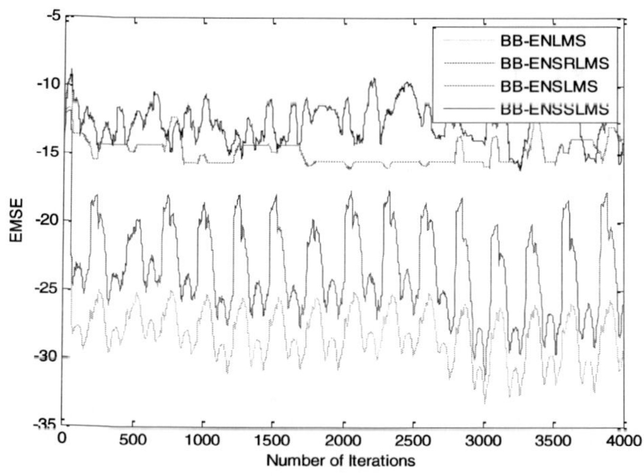

Figure 5.16. EMSE behavior in the PLI cancellation using block-based error nonlinear adaptive filtering techniques.

5.6.2. Adaptive Baseline Wander Removal

This experiment demonstrates BW cancellation, which is a non-stationary noise cancellation. The input to the filter is ECG signal is contaminated with respiration baseline wander; this is applied to a noise canceller shown in Figure 2.3. The reference signal is a real BW obtained from MIT-BIH Noise Stress Test Database. The contaminated ECG signal is applied as input $x(n) = s_1 + n_1$, the correlated noise reference is applied as n_2 and the output is y(n). Various filter structures are implemented using non-overlapping block filters BLMS, BNLMS, BENLMS, FBLMS, FBNLMS, FBENLMS and overlapping block filters BBNLMS, BBNSRLMS, BBNSLMS, BBNSSLMS, BBENLMS, BBENSRLMS, BBENSLMS and BBENSSLMS algorithms. The simulation results for adaptive BW removal using BLMS, its variants are shown in Figure 5.17 and Figure 5.18. The SNRI contrast for this case is shown in Table 5.6.

Figure 5.19 illustrates the results of the excess mean square error (EMSE) for BW reduction using BLMS and its variants in time, frequency domains. This phenomenon is also demonstrated in Table 5.12 and Table 5.13. The EMSE and M_{ad} are calculated for different types of artefacts over the data set considered and average values are taken.

Table 5.6 clears that FBENLMS efficiently reduces BW noise from ECG signals.

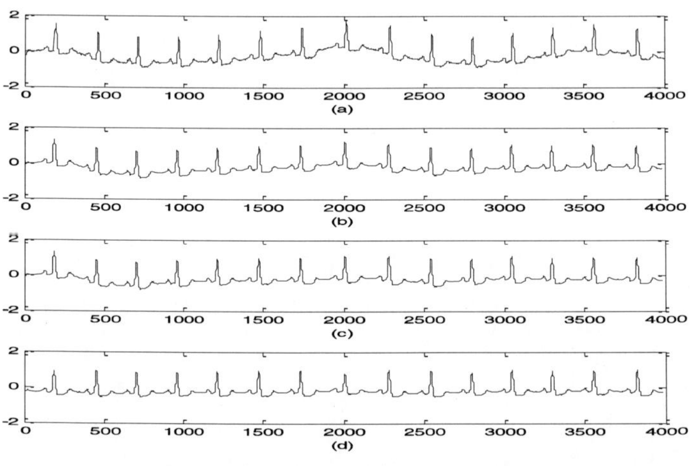

Figure 5.17. Typical filtering results for BW cancellation using BLMS and its variants in time domain: (a) ECG signal with BW, (b) recovered signal using BLMS algorithm, (c) recovered signal using BNLMS algorithm, (d) recovered signal using BENLMS algorithm.

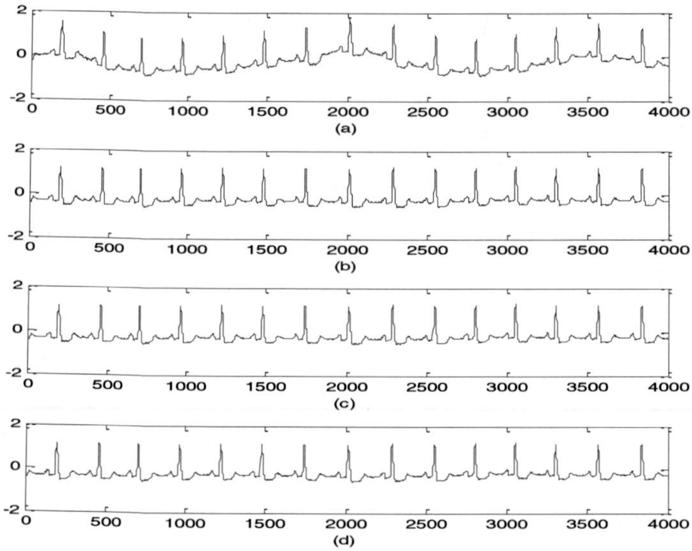

Figure 5.18. Typical filtering results for BW cancellation using FBLMS and its variants in frequency domain: (a) ECG signal with BW, (b) recovered signal using FBLMS algorithm, (c) recovered signal using FBNLMS algorithm, (d) recovered signal using FBENLMS algorithm.

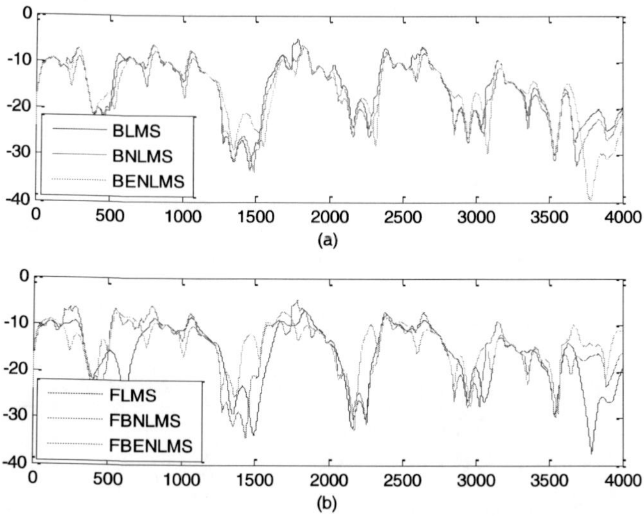

Figure 5.19. EMSE behavior in the BW cancellation using block adaptive filtering techniques.

Table 5.6. Performance contrast of block adaptive filters for the removal of BW

Rec. No.	BLMS	FBLMS	BNLMS	FBNLMS	BENLMS	FBENLMS
100	2.8495	17.1887	3.2244	17.9965	3.4687	19.1620
105	4.1451	12.5573	4.6531	13.5793	4.8626	14.7234
108	3.4977	17.5619	3.8502	18.6683	4.0609	19.4367
203	3.0328	15.6994	3.7641	16.3639	3.9350	16.9500
228	3.9258	16.3239	4.2813	17.2060	4.5633	18.3126
Average	3.4901	15.8662	3.9546	16.7628	4.1781	17.7085

The simulation results for adaptive BW removal using block based normalized algorithms and its signed versions are shown in Figure 5.20 and Figure 5.21. The SNRI contrast for this case is shown in Table 5.7. Figure 5.22 and Figure 5.23 illustrates the results of the EMSE for BW reduction using BBNLMS, BBENLMS and its sign-based versions.

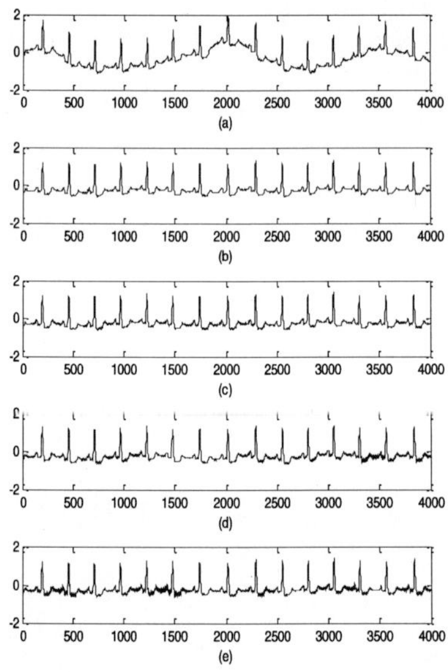

Figure 5.20. Typical filtering results for BW cancellation using block-based data normalized adaptive filtering techniques: (a) ECG signal with BW, (b) recovered signal using BBNLMS algorithm, (c) recovered signal using BBNSRLMS algorithm, (d) recovered signal using BBNSLMS algorithm, (e) recovered signal using BBNSSLMS algorithm.

Table 5.7. Performance contrast of block based normalized adaptive filters for the removal of BW

Rec. No.	BBNLMS	BBENLMS	BBNSRLMS	BBNSLMS	BBNSSLMS	BBENSRLMS	BBENSLMS	BBENSSLMS
100	9.5217	9.9582	7.4645	6.9348	4.9120	9.2336	6.5712	6.1158
105	11.9814	10.7641	9.3007	6.9696	6.2112	10.1198	7.3474	6.2850
108	10.7583	10.9378	6.7958	6.6014	5.2817	9.9423	7.2878	6.5932
203	9.8540	10.4481	7.0365	5.5887	4.8235	9.6287	7.6442	6.2184
228	11.2315	8.8435	8.4255	7.1900	6.2572	8.0898	7.1842	6.3216
Avg.	10.6693	10.1903	7.8046	6.6569	5.4971	9.4028	7.2069	6.3068

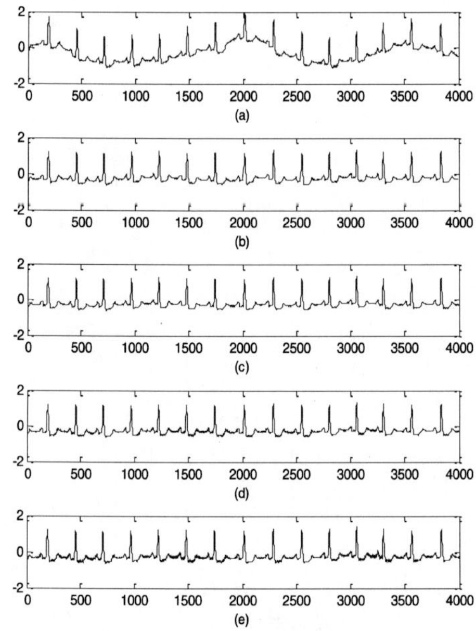

Figure 5.21. Typical filtering results for BW cancellation using block-based error nonlinear adaptive filtering techniques: (a) ECG signal with BW, (b) recovered signal using BBENLMS algorithm, (c) recovered signal using BBENSRLMS algorithm, (d) recovered signal using BBENSLMS algorithm, (e) recovered signal using BBENSSLMS algorithm.

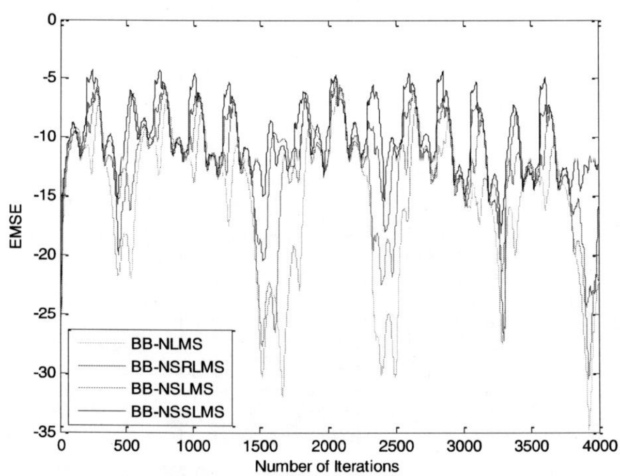

Figure 5.22. EMSE behavior in the BW cancellation using block-based data normalized adaptive filtering techniques.

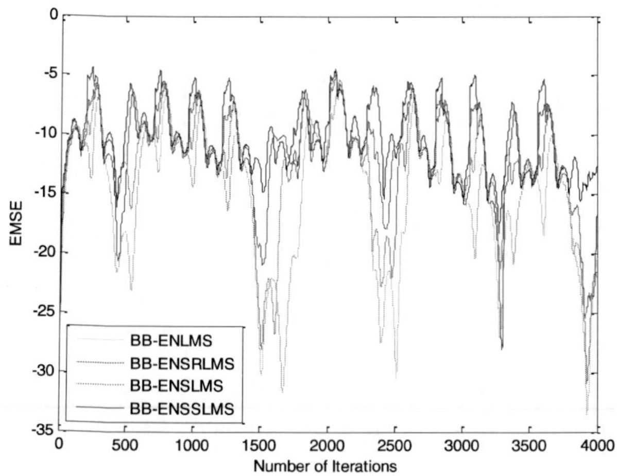

Figure 5.23. EMSE behavior in the BW cancellation using block-based error nonlinear adaptive filtering techniques.

This phenomenon is also demonstrated in Table 5.14 and Table 5.15. The EMSE and M_{ad} are calculated for different types of artefacts over the data set considered and average values are taken.

Table 5.7 gives the SNRI measurements for BW removal using block-based algorithms. Among these algorithms BBENSRLMS achieves highest SNRI with minimal complexity and then BBNSRLMS gets next place.

5.6.3. Adaptive Cancellation of Muscle Artefacts

This experiment demonstrates MA cancellation, which is a non-stationary noise cancellation. The input to the filter is ECG signal is contaminated with respiration baseline wander; this is applied to a noise canceller shown in Figure 2.3. The reference signal is a real MA obtained from MIT-BIH Noise Stress Test Database. The MA originally had a sampling frequency of 360Hz and therefore they were anti-alias re-sampled to 128Hz in order to match the sampling rate of the ECG. The contaminated ECG signal is applied as input $x(n) = s_1 + n_1$, the correlated noise reference is applied as n_2 and the output is $y(n)$. Various filter structures are implemented using non-overlapping block filters BLMS, BNLMS, BENLMS, FBLMS, FBNLMS, FBENLMS and overlapping block filters BBNLMS, BBNSRLMS, BBNSLMS, BBNSSLMS, BBENLMS, BBENSRLMS, BBENSLMS and BBENSSLMS algorithms. The simulation results for adaptive MA removal using BLMS, its variants are shown in Figure 5.24 and Figure 5.25. The SNRI contrast for this case is shown in Table 5.8. Figure 5.24 illustrates the results of the EMSE for MA reduction using BLMS and its variants in time, frequency domains. This phenomenon is also demonstrated in Table 5.12 and Table 5.13. The EMSE and M_{ad} are calculated for different types of artefacts over the data set considered and average values are taken using MATLAB programs.

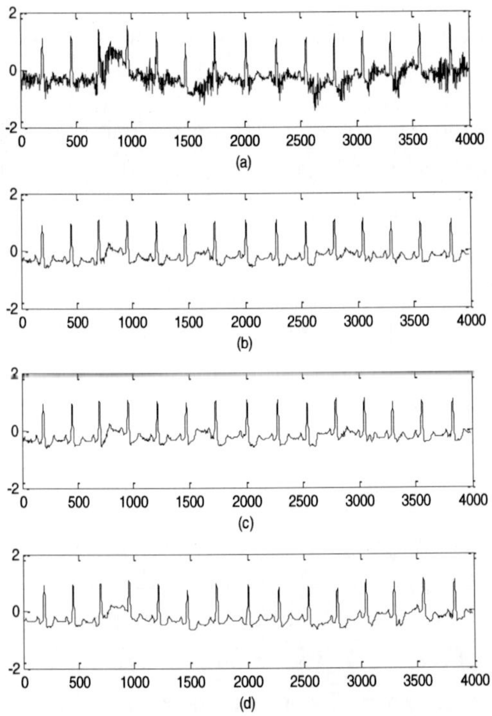

Figure 5.24. Typical filtering results for MA cancellation using BLMS and its variants in time domain: (a) ECG signal with MA, (b) recovered signal using BLMS algorithm, (c) recovered signal using BNLMS algorithm, (d) recovered signal using BENLMS algorithm.

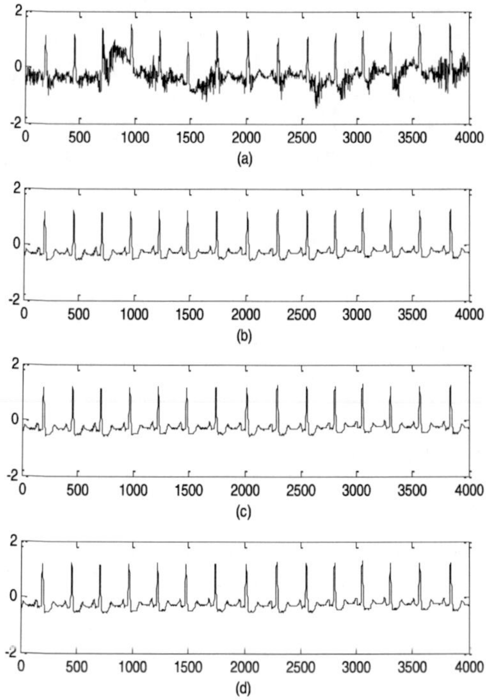

Figure 5.25. Typical filtering results for MA cancellation using FBLMS and its variants in frequency domain: (a) ECG signal with MA, (b) recovered signal using FBLMS algorithm, (c) recovered signal using FBNLMS algorithm, (d) recovered signal using FBENLMS algorithm.

Table 5.8. Performance contrast of block filters for the removal of MA

Rec. No.	BLMS	FBLMS	BNLMS	FBNLMS	BENLMS	FBENLMS
100	4.0578	17.1893	4.5530	17.7261	4.8765	18.2226
105	5.5495	12.5753	5.9850	13.4783	6.3850	14.5783
108	4.4197	17.7117	4.8840	17.7254	5.2561	18.8467
203	6.6705	15.9857	7.1768	17.1543	7.5648	18.1026
228	5.5143	16.3317	6.0197	16.9821	6.4723	18.3314
Average	5.2423	15.9587	5.7237	16.6132	6.1109	17.6163

Table 5.8 clearly shows that for the MA removal frequency domain filters performs efficiently. Among these FBENLMS achieves highest SNRI.

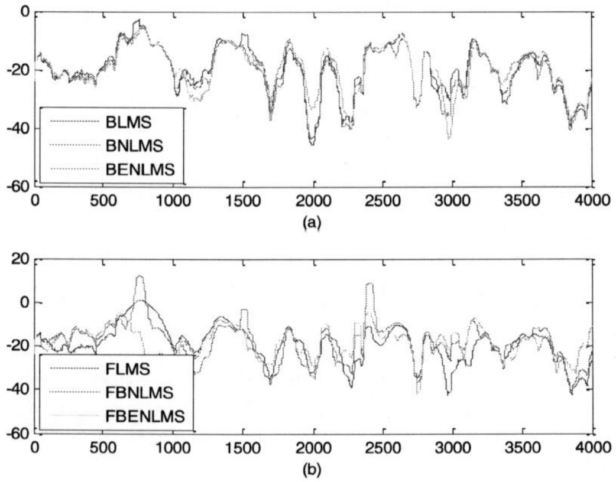

Figure 5.26. EMSE behavior in the MA cancellation using block adaptive filtering techniques.

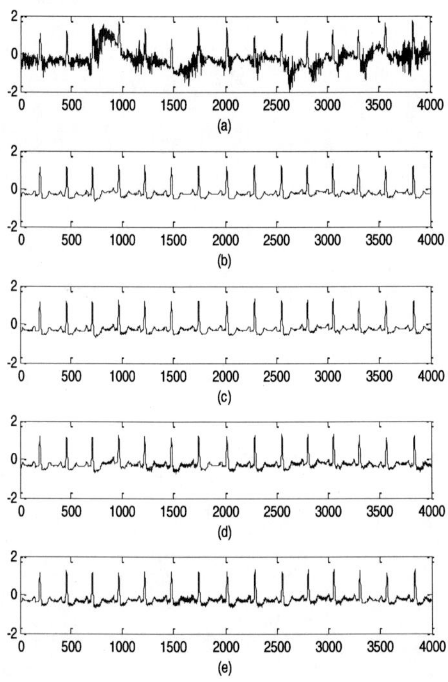

Figure 5.27. Typical filtering results for MA cancellation using block-based data normalized adaptive filtering techniques: (a) ECG signal with MA, (b) recovered signal using BBNLMS algorithm, (c) recovered signal using BBNSRLMS algorithm, (d) recovered signal using BBNSLMS algorithm, (e) recovered signal using BBNSSLMS algorithm.

Table 5.9. Performance contrast of block based normalized adaptive filters for the removal of MA

Rec. No.	BBNLMS	BBENLMS	BBNSRLMS	BBNSLMS	BBNSSLMS	BBENSRLMS	BBENSLMS	BBENSSLMS
100	9.4285	10.3754	6.7857	5.0863	4.5237	9.8890	8.3126	7.0525
105	11.9879	10.5279	9.6467	6.6011	4.8847	10.3752	8.2742	7.1625
108	10.3147	11.2148	7.7298	6.2130	5.5384	10.9672	8.2747	7.2396
203	12.0237	10.1925	9.4912	8.1992	7.0282	9.9364	9.0715	8.2501
228	10.1578	10.2768	8.6244	7.3276	6.5730	9.9789	8.4353	7.8064
Average	10.7825	10.5174	8.4555	6.6847	5.7096	10.2293	8.4736	7.5022

The performance of adaptive MA removal using block based normalized algorithms and its signed versions are shown in Figure 5.27 and Figure 5.28. The SNRI contrast for this case is shown in Table 5.8. Figure 5.29 and Figure 5.30 illustrates the results of the EMSE for MA reduction using BBNLMS, BBENLMS and its sign-based versions. This phenomenon is also demonstrated in Table 5.14 and Table 5.15. The EMSE and M_{ad} are calculated for different types of artefacts over the data set considered and average values are taken.

From Table 5.9 it is clear that among all block-based algorithms, BBENSRLMS achieves highest SNRI with minimal computational complexity in the cancellation of MA noise.

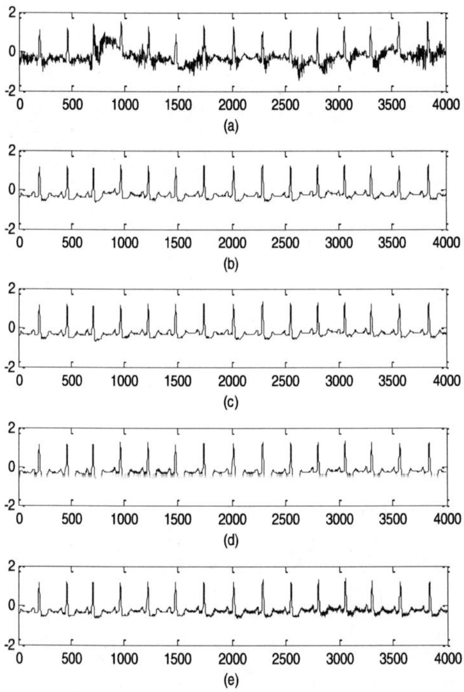

Figure 5.28. Typical filtering results for MA cancellation using block-based error nonlinear adaptive filtering techniques: (a) ECG signal with MA, (b) recovered signal using BBENLMS algorithm, (c) recovered signal using BBENSRLMS algorithm, (d) recovered signal using BBENSLMS algorithm, (e) recovered signal using BBENSSLMS algorithm.

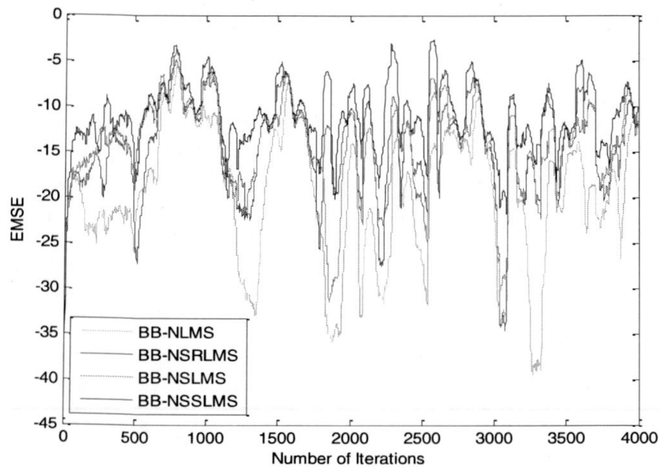

Figure 5.29. EMSE behavior in the MA cancellation using block-based data normalized adaptive filtering techniques.

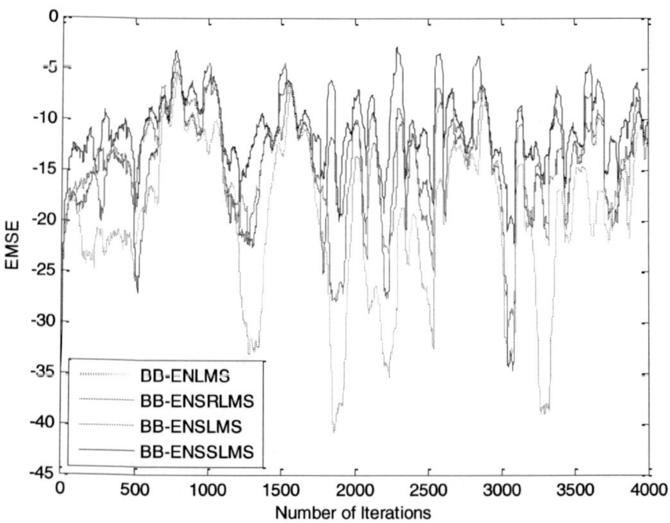

Figure 5.30. EMSE behavior in the MA cancellation using block-based error nonlinear adaptive filtering techniques.

5.6.4. Adaptive Cancellation of Electrode Motion Artefacts

This experiment demonstrates EM cancellation, which is a non-stationary noise cancellation. The input to the filter is ECG signal is contaminated with respiration baseline wander; this is applied to a noise canceller shown in Figure 2.3. The reference signal is a real EM obtained from MIT-BIH Noise Stress Test Database. The EM originally had a sampling frequency of 360Hz and therefore they were anti-alias re-sampled to 128Hz in order to match the sampling rate of the ECG. Various filter structures are implemented using non-overlapping block filters BLMS, BNLMS, BENLMS, FBLMS, FBNLMS, FBENLMS and overlapping block filters BBNLMS, BBNSRLMS, BBNSLMS, BBNSSLMS, BBENLMS, BBENSRLMS, BBENSLMS and BBENSSLMS algorithms. The simulation results for adaptive EM removal using BLMS, its variants are shown in Figure 5.31 and Figure 5.32. The SNRI contrast for this case is shown in Table 5.10. Figure 5.33 illustrates the results of the EMSE for EM reduction using BLMS and its variants in time, frequency domains. This phenomenon is also demonstrated in Table 5.12 and Table 5.13. The EMSE and M_{ad} are calculated for different types of artefacts over the data set considered and average values are taken.

Table 5.10 shows the performance block adaptive filters in time domain and frequency domain, it clears that frequency domain filters enhances ECG signals efficiently. In the EM removal FBENLMS filters efficiently.

The performance of adaptive EM removal using block based normalized algorithms and its signed versions are shown in Figure 5.34 and Figure 5.35. The SNRI contrast for this case is shown in Table 5.11. Figure 5.36 and Figure 5.37 illustrates the results of the EMSE for EM reduction using BBNLMS, BBENLMS and its sign-based versions. This phenomenon is also demonstrated in Table 5.14 and Table 5.15. The EMSE and M_{ad} are calculated for different types of artefacts over the data set considered and average values are taken.

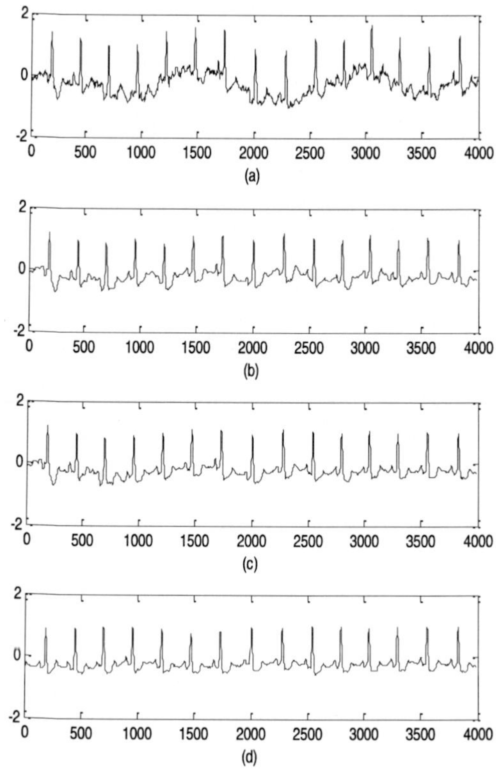

Figure 5.31. Typical filtering results for EM cancellation using BLMS and its variants in time domain: (a) ECG signal with EM, (b) recovered signal using BLMS algorithm, (c) recovered signal using BNLMS algorithm, (d) recovered signal using BENLMS algorithm.

Table 5.10. Performance contrast of block adaptive filters for the removal of EM

Rec. No.	BLMS	FBLMS	BNLMS	FBNLMS	BENLMS	FBENLMS
100	3.3750	17.2193	3.8248	17.9561	4.1050	18.7227
105	4.4273	12.5753	4.7919	13.3706	4.9835	14.5783
108	3.4879	17.7117	3.9150	18.6114	4.2143	19.3172
203	3.7391	15.9857	4.0235	16.7704	4.3670	17.6019
228	4.0565	16.3310	4.4840	17.1321	5.0255	18.3314
Average	3.8171	15.9646	4.2078	16.7681	4.5390	17.7103

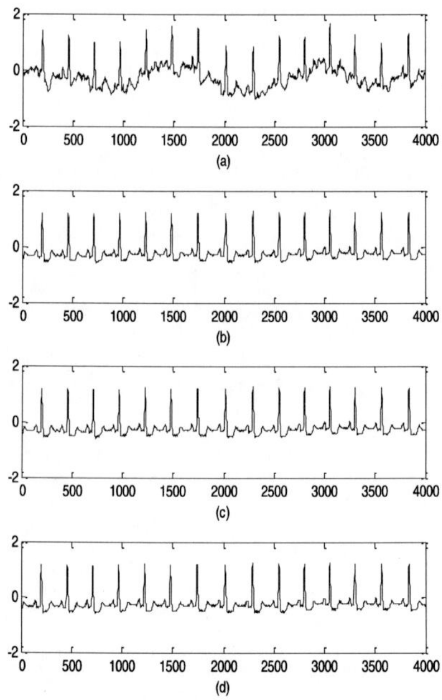

Figure 5.32. Typical filtering results for EM cancellation using BLMS and its variants in frequency domain: (a) ECG signal with EM, (b) recovered signal using FBLMS algorithm, (c) recovered signal using FBNLMS algorithm, (d) recovered signal using FBENLMS algorithm.

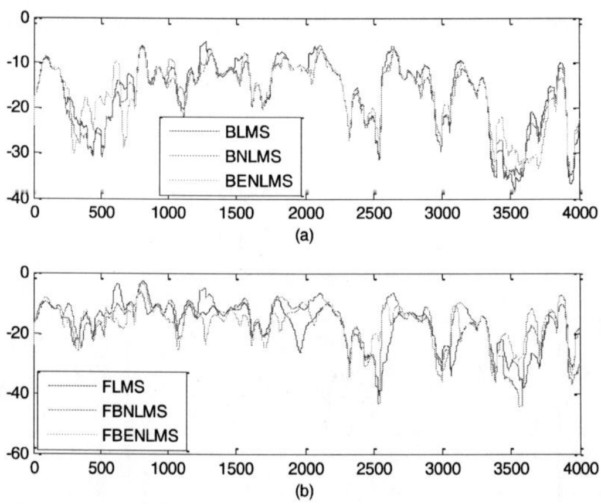

Figure 5.33. EMSE behavior in the EM cancellation using block adaptive filtering techniques.

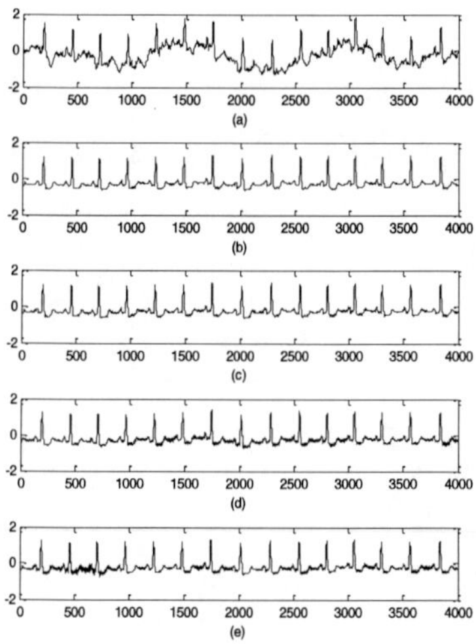

Figure 5.34. Typical filtering results for EM cancellation using block-based data normalized adaptive filtering techniques: (a) ECG signal with EM, (b) recovered signal using BBNLMS algorithm, (c) recovered signal using BBNSRLMS algorithm, (d) recovered signal using BBNSLMS algorithm, (e) recovered signal using BBNSSLMS algorithm.

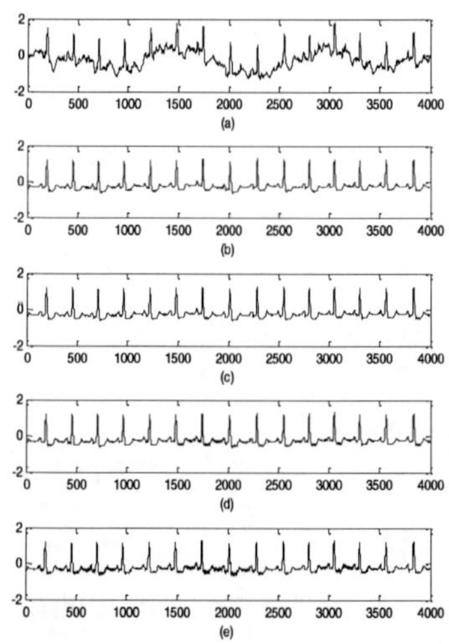

Figure 5.35. Typical filtering results for EM cancellation using block-based error nonlinear adaptive filtering techniques: (a) ECG signal with EM, (b) recovered signal using BBENLMS algorithm, (c) recovered signal using BBENSRLMS algorithm, (d) recovered signal using BBENSLMS algorithm, (e) recovered signal using BBENSSLMS algorithm.

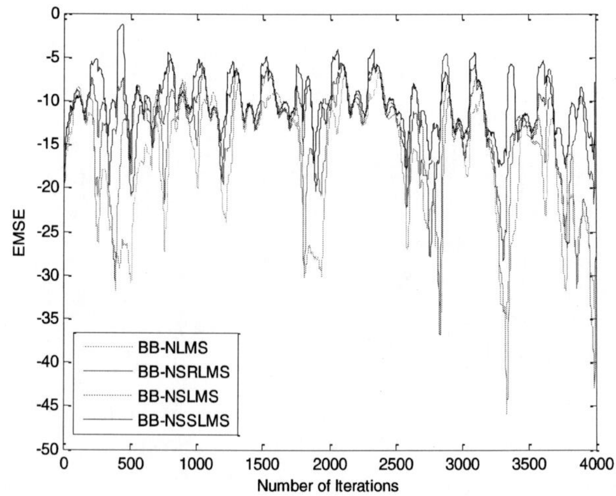

Figure 5.36. EMSE behavior in the EM cancellation using block-based data normalized adaptive filtering techniques.

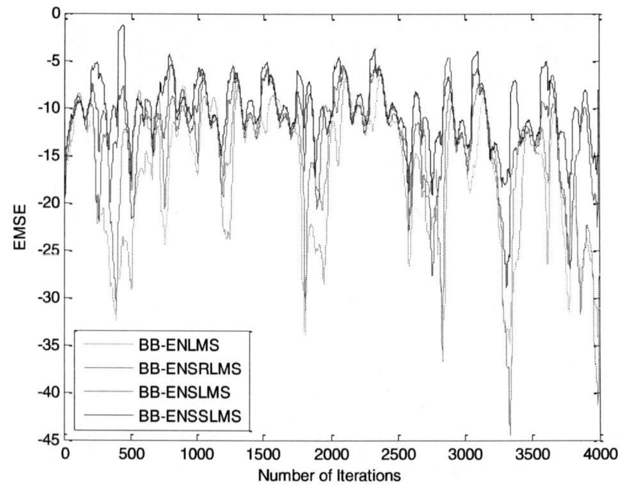

Figure 5.37. EMSE behavior in the EM cancellation using block-based error nonlinear adaptive filtering techniques.

From Table 5.11 it is clear that in EM cancellation BBENSRLMS gets highest SNRI with minimal computational complexity and BBNSRLMS gets next place.

Table 5.11. Performance contrast of block based normalized adaptive filters for the removal of EM

Rec. No.	BBNLMS	BBENLMS	BBNSRLMS	BBNSLMS	BBNSSLMS	BBENSRLMS	BBENSLMS	BBENSSLMS
100	11.2869	10.6754	8.9416	6.3333	5.6090	10.3052	7.3792	6.8510
105	12.9843	11.8975	10.2849	7.8379	6.8032	11.5198	8.4284	6.9918
108	11.4761	10.7694	8.0243	6.0553	5.5755	10.4126	7.0929	6.0526
203	10.9875	10.2571	7.6493	6.7010	5.9975	9.9974	7.8728	7.9222
228	10.9531	10.1694	7.6063	6.7485	6.2828	9.6592	7.3895	6.1434
Average	11.5375	10.7537	8.5012	6.7352	6.0536	10.3788	7.6325	6.7922

Table 5.12. A comparison of EMSE and M_{ad} for various artefacts using BLMS, BNLMS and BENLMS algorithms in time domain

Noise Type	Record Number	BLMS		BNLMS		BENLMS	
		EMSE	M_{ad}	EMSE	M_{ad}	EMSE	M_{ad}
PLI	100	-23.5158	0.0338	-37.6045	0.0013	-38.5890	0.0011
	105	-26.9485	0.0139	-37.3315	0.0013	-37.8000	0.0011
	108	-23.4555	0.0370	-37.6604	0.0014	-37.3595	0.0015
	203	-28.7802	0.0051	-36.2603	0.0009	-37.6502	0.0006
	228	-27.5581	0.0178	-37.9004	0.0016	-38.2507	0.0015
	Average	**-26.0516**	**0.0215**	**-37.3514**	**0.0013**	**-37.9298**	**0.0011**
BW	100	-8.8100	0.9998	-12.0405	0.4752	-11.7290	0.5105
	105	-11.2375	0.5172	-12.2016	0.3687	-13.8071	0.3203
	108	-8.8284	1.0746	-12.3452	0.4882	-12.2886	0.4744
	203	-8.1492	0.3922	-11.6411	0.2828	-11.6130	0.2657
	228	-10.0960	0.9901	-13.9642	0.4063	-13.7003	0.4317
	Average	**-9.4242**	**0.7947**	**-12.4385**	**0.4042**	**-12.6276**	**0.4005**

Table 5.12. (Continued)

Noise Type	Record Number	BLMS		BNLMS		BENLMS	
		EMSE	M_{ad}	EMSE	EMSE	M_{ad}	EMSE
MA	100	-12.1000	0.4687	-14.5195	0.3686	-14.6068	0.3001
	105	-13.0003	0.3447	-15.3892	0.2288	-14.9090	0.2369
	108	-11.3294	0.6042	-14.1812	0.3133	-14.2485	0.3085
	203	-10.2375	0.9287	-12.5340	0.2149	-12.8756	0.1987
	228	-13.7342	0.4403	-15.5322	0.2787	-16.9366	0.2049
	Average	**-12.0808**	**0.5573**	**-14.4312**	**0.2808**	**-14.7153**	**0.2498**
EM	100	-8.5646	0.8714	-12.7274	0.4057	-12.2474	0.4531
	105	-10.7450	0.5602	-13.5392	0.3044	-13.9778	0.2909
	108	-10.5723	0.4789	-12.5324	0.4580	-12.5811	0.4529
	203	-9.4849	0.4337	-10.6291	0.3350	-11.2857	0.2865
	228	-8.2993	0.8437	-13.9422	0.4084	-13.6013	0.4415
	Average	**-9.5332**	**0.3675**	**-12.6740**	**0.3823**	**-12.7386**	**0.3849**

Table 5.13. A comparison of EMSE and M_{ad} for various artefacts using BLMS, BNLMS and BENLMS algorithms in frequency domain

Noise Type	Record Number	FBLMS		FBNLMS		FBENLMS	
		EMSE	M_{ad}	EMSE	M_{ad}	EMSE	M_{ad}
PLI	100	-33.7909	0.0032	-35.3008	0.0022	-32.0525	0.0047
	105	-35.2056	0.0021	-36.2671	0.0016	-31.2780	0.0051
	108	-36.6369	0.0018	-36.7086	0.0018	-30.0221	0.0082
	203	-31.0637	0.0030	-33.6735	0.0017	-31.4613	0.0028
	228	-31.3464	0.0074	-36.5536	0.0022	-36.7641	0.0021
	Average	**-33.6087**	**0.0035**	**-35.7007**	**0.0019**	**-32.3156**	**0.0045**
BW	100	-8.9598	0.9905	-10.2087	0.7245	-12.0130	0.4782
	105	-8.7653	1.0526	-12.3540	0.4000	-13.0967	0.3371
	108	-9.6381	0.9627	-10.6515	0.7062	-13.3298	0.3812
	203	-8.0328	1.5219	-12.6948	0.2450	-15.8150	0.1010
	228	-8.2790	0.9989	-11.8263	0.6647	-12.6820	0.5458
	Average	**-8.7350**	**1.1053**	**-11.5470**	**0.5480**	**-13.3873**	**0.3686**
MA	100	-9.0992	0.9369	-12.8683	0.3127	-13.4866	0.2771
	105	-8.4714	1.4563	-13.7531	0.2898	-12.1918	0.5226
	108	-10.1964	0.7122	-13.1162	0.4004	-14.6660	0.2802
	203	-8.6603	0.5244	-12.5601	0.2136	-14.2519	0.1447
	228	-8.6645	1.7366	-14.9567	0.3233	-15.0598	0.2974
	Average	**-9.0183**	**1.0012**	**-13.4508**	**0.3079**	**-13.9312**	**0.3044**
EM	100	-9.3916	0.8745	-11.4686	0.5421	-12.4491	0.4325
	105	-11.1320	0.3993	-13.7890	0.2874	-13.9568	0.2335
	108	-11.0551	0.5912	-12.7695	0.5459	-14.5256	0.2844
	203	-9.9990	0.3853	-10.0071	0.3845	-14.6932	0.1307
	228	-8.6419	0.9742	-12.8987	0.5193	-14.4739	0.3613
	Average	**-10.0439**	**0.6449**	**-12.1065**	**0.4558**	**-14.0197**	**0.2884**

Table 5.14. A comparison of EMSE and M_{ad} for various artifacts using block-based data normalized algorithms

Noise Type	Record Number	BBNLMS		BBNSRLMS		BBNSLMS		BBNSSLMS	
		EMSE	M_{ad}	EMSE	M_{ad}	EMSE	M_{ad}	EMSE	M_{ad}
PLI	100	-28.5849	0.0105	-25.8085	0.0200	-12.6174	0.4161	-12.3809	0.4394
	105	-28.5900	0.0095	-25.6457	0.0187	-14.5399	0.2418	-13.4632	0.3098
	108	-28.7732	0.0109	-26.2020	0.0197	-13.3219	0.3819	-13.0330	0.4081
	203	-26.2273	0.0092	-23.0210	0.0192	-15.3475	0.1124	-13.6814	0.1650
	228	-29.7644	0.0107	-26.8872	0.0207	-13.4669	0.4556	-13.0324	0.5035
	Average	**-28.3879**	**0.0101**	**-25.5128**	**0.0196**	**-13.8587**	**0.3215**	**-13.1181**	**0.3651**
BW	100	-11.3769	0.5536	-9.9424	0.7703	-10.0876	0.7450	-9.2732	0.8987
	105	-12.3414	0.3929	-10.1133	0.6700	-10.9681	0.5503	-8.9405	0.8448
	108	-11.4001	0.5944	-10.0770	0.8061	-10.1874	0.7859	-9.4730	0.9264
	203	-9.9203	0.3923	-707570	0.6456	-8.5665	0.5358	-6.5823	0.8461
	228	-12. 7764	0.5341	-11.0836	0.7887	-11.2854	0.7529	-10.2255	0.9610
	Average	**-11.5810**	**0.4934**	**-9.7946**	**0.7361**	**-10.2190**	**0.6739**	**-8.8989**	**0.9020**
MA	100	-14.1028	0.2956	-11.3597	0.5558	-11.8046	0.5017	-8.5944	1.0507
	105	-15.1616	0.2095	-1108460	0.4496	-12.1778	0.4165	-9.4898	0.7735
	108	-13.8748	0.3362	-11.2722	0.6122	-12.0010	0.5176	-9.3823	0.9460
	203	-12.5593	0.2137	-9.7898	0.4043	-10.7110	0.3270	-7.7307	0.6495
	228	-15.9790	0.2555	-12.7685	0.5351	-13.2730	0.4764	-10.1459	0.9788
	Average	**-14.3355**	**0.2621**	**-11.4072**	**0.5114**	**-11.9934**	**0.4478**	**-9.6686**	**0.8797**
EM	100	-11.9675	0.4833	-10.3399	0.7030	-10.4484	0.6856	-9.2794	0.8974
	105	-13.1557	0.3326	-10.3940	0.6281	-11.5321	0.4833	-8.8689	0.8924
	108	-12.0457	0.5123	-10.2951	0.7666	-10.8610	0.6730	-9.3711	0.9484
	203	-9.7166	0.4112	-7.6287	0.6650	-8.4345	0.5523	-6.6213	0.8386
	228	-13.7103	0.4308	-11.6962	0.6849	-12.2369	0.6047	-10.1557	0.9765
	Average	**-12.1191**	**0.4340**	**-10.0707**	**0.6897**	**-10.7025**	**0.5997**	**-8.8792**	**0.9106**

Table 5.15. A comparison of EMSE and M_{ad} for various artifacts using block-based error nonlinear algorithms

Noise Type	Record Number	BBENLMS		BBENSRLMS		BBENSLMS		BBENSSLMS	
		EMSE	M_{ad}	EMSE	M_{ad}	EMSE	M_{ad}	EMSE	M_{ad}
PLI	100	-27.3062	0.0141	-22.7218	0.0406	-13.9239	0.3080	-12.0563	0.4735
	105	-27.9371	0.0111	-22.4143	0.0394	-14.8008	0.2277	-12.4178	0.3941
	108	-28.0491	0.0129	-22.4193	0.0470	-13.8203	0.3405	-12.1524	0.4999
	203	-26.9338	0.0078	-30.7420	0.0032	-23.2544	0.0182	-21.1764	0.0294
	228	-28.4237	0.0146	-24.1106	0.0393	-15.1117	0.3120	-12.5275	0.5656
	Average	**-27.7299**	**0.0121**	**-24.4810**	**0.0339**	**-16.1822**	**0.2412**	**-14.0660**	**0.3925**
BW	100	-11.2302	0.5727	-10.0043	0.7594	-10.1475	0.7348	-9.3821	0.8764
	105	-12.3441	0.4009	-10.1900	0.6583	-10.9514	0.5524	-9.1478	0.8369
	108	-11.4477	0.5879	-10.0835	0.8049	-10.2291	0.7784	-9.4292	0.9358
	203	-10.1430	0.3727	-9.7945	0.4038	-10.2020	0.3677	-8.3473	0.5636
	228	-12.6911	0.5447	-11.1476	0.7771	-11.3502	0.7417	-10.2907	0.9467
	Average	**-11.5712**	**0.4957**	**-10.2439**	**0.6807**	**-10.3760**	**0.6356**	**-9.3194**	**0.8318**
MA	100	-13.8930	0.3102	-11.3886	0.5522	-11.6943	0.5146	-8.6106	1.0468
	105	-15.0772	0.2136	-11.8231	0.4520	-12.0463	0.4293	-9.3440	0.7999
	108	-13.9682	0.3291	-11.3181	0.6057	-11.9942	0.5184	-9.3653	0.9497
	203	-13.1442	0.1867	-11.1967	0.2924	-12.2429	0.2298	-9.1699	0.4663
	228	-15.9399	0.2578	-12.7901	0.5324	-13.3003	0.4734	-10.0616	0.9979
	Average	**-14.4045**	**0.2594**	**-11.7033**	**0.4869**	**-12.2555**	**0.4331**	**-9.3102**	**0.8521**
EM	100	-11.8437	0.4972	-10.3641	0.6991	-10.4511	0.6852	-9.2820	0.8969
	105	-13.1871	0.3302	-10.4643	0.6180	-11.5155	0.4852	-8.8731	0.8915
	108	-12.1404	0.5013	-10.3093	0.7641	-10.8632	0.6726	-9.3341	0.9565
	203	-10.1767	0.3698	-9.0751	0.4766	-10.0560	0.3802	-7.5470	0.6776
	228	-13.6404	0.4377	-11.8152	0.6664	-12.3057	0.5952	-10.3616	0.9313
	Average	**-12.1976**	**0.4277**	**-10.4056**	**0.6448**	**-11.0383**	**0.5636**	**-9.0795**	**0.8707**

From Tables 5.12, 5.13 it is clear that lower EMSE and M_{ad} are achieved in frequency domain filtering. However, these values are lower for tome domain algorithms also, due to signal averaging in weight updating process, the amplitude of the signals in time domain decreases, as a result the SNRI in time domain case is lower than frequency domain even though time domain algorithms achieves comparable EMSE and M_{ad}. Similarly, Tables 5.14, 5.15 shows EMSE and M_{ad} for overlapping block-based filters. Here BBNLMS and BBENLMS get lower values but the computational complexity is large. BBENSRLMS and BBNSRLMS gets EMSE and M_{ad} comparable to BBNLMS and BBENLMS with single multiplication to compute weight update recursion, so these filters are preferable.

5.7. CONCLUSION

In this chapter the problem of noise cancelation from ECG signal using overlapping block and non-overlapping block adaptive filters are developed and tested on real signals with different artefacts obtained from the MIT-BIH database.

We have developed adaptive filters using BLMS algorithm. The convergence characteristics of BLMS are approximately similar to that of LMS algorithm. However due to signal averaging the amplitude of the ECG signal reduces, this leads to low SNR. In order to improve convergence rate and filtering capability we applied normalization to block adaptive filters. Here data normalization and error normalization are considered. This result BNLMS algorithm and BENLMS algorithm. From our experiments it is clear that normalization improves filtering capability. These block algorithms are also implemented in frequency domain viz., FBLMS, FBNLMS and FBENLMS algorithms. Frequency domain treatment improves the resolution and SNRI.

We also developed overlapping block-based ANCs for ECG denoising. The algorithms discussed in Chapter 4 are processed by overlapping block processing. These are BBNLMS and BBENLMS. In order to reduce computational complexity, we have successfully developed various ANCs using sign-based versions of both BBNLMS and BBENLMS. Between BBNLMS and BBENLMS the performance of BBNLMS is found to be better in terms of SNRI, EMSE and M. Among the six sign-based algorithms BBNSRLMS got first place, next goes to BBENSRLMS and then BBNSLMS, BBNSSLMS, BBENSLMS, BBENSSLMS in the descending order. From the simulation results it is clear that the proposed ANCs remove non-stationary noise efficiently. The proposed treatment provides high signal to noise ratio with less computational complexity. Hence the sign-based algorithms are more suitable in wireless biotelemetry ECG systems.

Therefore, in this chapter totally we have developed six non-overlapping ANCs and eight overlapping ANCs for ECG denoising. Among the ANCs FBNLMS, FBENLMS, BBNSRLMS and BBENSRLMS are performing better that other, so these are considered for development on digital signal processor in real time environment.

5.8. Review of Simulation Studies

In Chapter 3 we have developed five LMS based ANCs using weight update variants of LMS algorithm namely Leaky LMS, Dead zone LMS, LMF and Median LMS algorithms. Among the five LMS based algorithms DZLMS and LMF algorithms performs better in the non-stationary noise removal. To reduce the computational complexity, we combine these five algorithms with sign regressor algorithm, sign algorithm and sign sign algorithm, results fifteen algorithms. Among the sign-based versions the SRLMS, SRLLMS, DZSRLMS, SRLMF, SRMLMS algorithms performs better with respect to convergence, SNRI, EMSE measurement, misadjustment and computational complexity. All the remaining SA and SSA based ANCs are slightly inferior to their LMS counterpart. Therefore, totally twenty ANCs are developed in this chapter.

In Chapter 4, we have developed two types of normalized filters i.e., data normalized, error normalized and their signed based versions, totally eight ANCs are developed for ECG denoising. Among six sign-based algorithms NSRLMS got first place, next goes to ENSRLMS and then NSLMS, NSSLMS, ENSLMS, ENSSLMS in the descending order. The filtering performance of all these algorithms is better than LMS algorithm, whereas the number of multiplications is less than that of LMS except one division operation is needed for normalization. In this chapter totally eight ANCs are developed.

In Chapter 5, we have developed non-overlapping and overlapping block adaptive filters. In non-overlapping category BLMS, BNLMS, BENLMS and their frequency domain versions FBLMS, FBNLMS, FBENLMS based ANCs are developed for ECG enhancement. In overlapping category, we developed BBNLMS, BBENLMS and their six sign-based algorithms i.e., BBNSRLMS, BBNSLMS, BBNSSLMS, BBENSRLMS, BBENSLMS, BBENSSLMS algorithms. Fourteen ANCs are developed in this chapter. Therefore, totally forty-two adaptive noise cancellers for ECG denoising are developed.

These algorithms are listed below:

1. Least Mean Square (LMS) algorithm
2. Leaky Least Mean Square (LLMS) algorithm
3. Dead Zone Least Mean Square (DZLMS) algorithm
4. Least Mean Fourth (LMF) algorithm
5. Median Least Mean Square (MLMS) algorithm
6. Sign Regressor LMS (SRLMS) algorithm
7. Sign LMS (SLMS) algorithm
8. Sign Sign LMS (SSLMS) algorithm
9. Sign Regressor Leaky LMS (SRLLMS) algorithm
10. Sign Leaky LMS (SLLMS) algorithm
11. Sign Sign Leaky LMS (SSLLMS) algorithm
12. Sign Regressor Dead Zone LMS (SRDZLMS) algorithm
13. Sign Dead Zone LMS (SDZLMS) algorithm
14. Sign Sign Dead Zone LMS (SSDZLMS) algorithm
15. Sign Regressor LMF (SRLMF) algorithm
16. Sign LMF (SLMF) algorithm

17. Sign Sign LMF (SSLMF) algorithm
18. Sign Regressor Median LMS (SRMLMS) algorithm
19. Sign Median LMS (SMLMS) algorithm
20. Sign Sign Median LMS (SSMLMS) algorithm
21. Normalized LMS (NLMS) algorithm
22. Error nonlinear LMS (ENLMS) algorithm
23. Normalized Sign Regressor (NSRLMS) algorithm
24. Normalized Sign (NSLMS) algorithm
25. Normalized Sign Sign (NSSLMS) algorithm
26. Error nonlinear Sign Regressor LMS (ENSRLMS) algorithm
27. Error nonlinear Sign LMS (ENSLMS) algorithm
28. Error nonlinear Sign Sign LMS (ENSSLMS) algorithm
29. Block LMS (BLMS) algorithm
30. Block Normalized LMS (BNLMS) algorithm
31. Block Error nonlinear LMS (BENLMS) algorithm
32. Fast Block LMS (FBLMS) algorithm
33. Fast Block Normalized LMS (FBNLMS) algorithm
34. Fast Block Error nonlinear LMS (FBENLMS) algorithm
35. Block Based NLMS (BBNLMS) algorithm
36. Block Based Error nonlinear (BBENLMS) algorithm
37. Block Based NSRLMS (BBNSRLMS) algorithm
38. Block Based NSLMS (BBNSLMS) algorithm
39. Block Based NSSLMS (BBNSSLMS) algorithm
40. Block Based ESRLMS (BBESRLMS) algorithm
41. Block Based ESLMS (BBESLMS) algorithm
42. Block Based ESSLMS (BBESSLMS) algorithm

Among the algorithms from Chapter 3 DZSRLMS filters any of PLI, BW, MA, EM artefacts efficiently, it needs only one multiplication for computing the weight update recursion. SRLMS algorithm also filters with a SNRI closed to its unsigned realization. However, in impulsive environment when PLI is present LLMS and MLMS performs better than other, where as in SRA versions of LMS based algorithms the SNRI is close to their LMS counterpart. In the case of BW noise DZLMS and LMF performs better than other, in their signed versions SRDZLMS performs better than other algorithms. In MA cancellation LMF and DZLMS filters muscle artefacts efficiently, by achieving high SNRI, in the signed versions also these two achieves good SNRI, however SRLMF needs three multiplications and SRDZLMS need only one multiplication. In EM removal again LMF and DZLMS performs better than others, in the signed versions also these two achieves good SNRI.

In Chapter 4 NSRLMS and ENSRLMS removes artefacts in ECG signals efficiently with a smaller number of computations than LMS algorithm.

In Chapter 5 block processing-based frequency domain algorithms namely, FLMS, FBNLMS and FENLMS achieves highest SNRI i.e., frequency domain treatment increases the signal resolution, where as their time domain versions achieves better SNRI than LMS. In the case of overlapping block processing BBNSRLMS and BBENSRLMS achieves highest SNRI than the other overlapped block-based algorithms for all the four types of the artefacts considered.

Therefore, based on these considerations we choose SRDZLMS, SRLMS, NSRLMS, ENSRLMS, FBNLMS, FBENLMS, BBNSRLMS and BBENSRLMS for real time implementation on digital signal processor. For standardization LMS is considered for implementation.

Chapter 6

Implementation of Adaptive Filtering Techniques for the Removal of Noise in ECG Signals on Digital Signal Processor Based Embedded System

6.1. Introduction

In order to obtain high resolution ECG signals in real time environment, the noise canceller has to be developed on an embedded processor. Among various embedded processors like microprocessors, microcontrollers and digital signal processors (DSP) in real time development of signal processing algorithms DSP represent a key role. DSPs can handle different tasks, since they can be reprogrammed readily for a different application. R. Chassaing [118] states that DSPs can also perform the tasks in parallel instead of serial in case of traditional microprocessors. The digital signal processors have been very successful because of the development of software and hardware support. The following are the advantages of DSPs over the other processors [118],

- Can implement complex linear or nonlinear algorithms.
- Can modify easily by changing software.
- Reduced parts count makes fabrication easier.
- High reliability.

Some important features of DSPs to facilitate them for signal processing applications are,

1. Multiplication and Accumulations (MAC) and Multiple execution units: MACs operations are useful as the DSP applications typically have very high computational requirements in comparison to other types of computing tasks, since DSP algorithms in real time often must execute lengthy segments of signals with thousands of samples.
2. Efficient Memory Access: DSPs are facilitated with a feature of efficient memory access i.e., the ability to complete several accesses to memory in a single instruction cycle.
3. Circular Buffering: The need of processing the digital signals in real time, where the output has to be produced at the same time at which the input samples are being acquired, evolves the concept of circular buffering. Circular buffers are used to store the most recent values of a continuously updated signal.
4. Dedicated Address Generation Unit: This unit helps speed up the performance of the arithmetic processing on DSP. Once an appropriated addressing registers have been configured, the address generation unit operates in the background.
5. Specialized Instruction Sets: The instruction sets of the DSPs are designed to make maximum use of the processor's resources and at the same time minimize the memory space required to store the instructions. Some of the latest processors use very long instruction word (VLIW) architectures, where in multiple instructions are issued and executed per cycle.

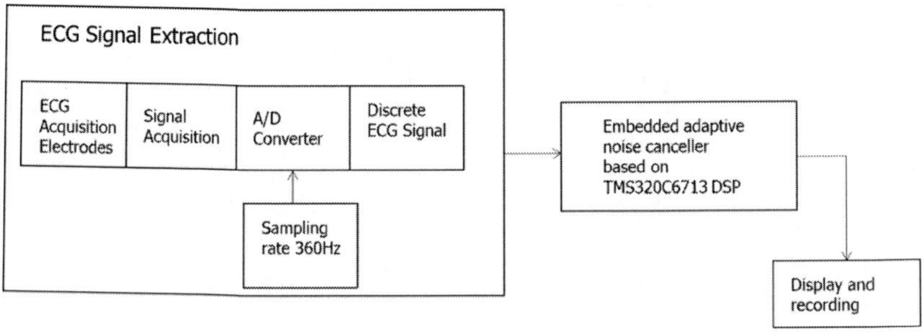

Figure. 6.1. Block diagram of ECG adaptive noise canceller developed on DSP.

We have therefore chosen a DSP as our embedded platform for the experimental verification of the developed adaptive noise cancellers in a real time environment. A generalized block diagram for ECG enhancement on DSP is shown in Figure 6.1. In the signal extraction chain, the signal is obtained from the patient using electrodes before undergoing analog to digital conversion with a 360 Hz sampling frequency. Discrete levels of various sample values now represent the ECG signal data. Our signals were obtained from the MIT-BIH data base [110]-[112], [161]-[162]. The ANC algorithms are developed and linked to the DSP and the filtered high-resolution ECG signals are recorded, displayed for diagnosis and immediate action.

To choose a suitable processor, we performed a literature study of various processors manufactured by different companies. These are listed below.

1. Analog devices [165]
2. Texas Instruments [166]
3. Freescale Semiconductors Inc [167]
4. Hyperstone DSP Processors [168]
5. VeriSilicon [169]

A comparison study of various DSPs from these companies is tabulated in Table 6.1.

Table 6.1. Comparison of various digital signal processors

S. No	Manufacturer	Processor Model	Fixed/ floating	Bus width	No. of Cores	VLIW	Memory	Clock frequency
1.	Analog Devices [165]	ADSP 21991 [170]	Fixed	16 bits	Single	Not supporting	32K Program Memory RAM, 8K Data Memory RAM	160MHz
2.	Analog Devices [165]	ADSP 21992 [171]	Fixed	16 bits	Single	Not supporting	32K Program Memory RAM, 16K Data Memory RAM	160MHz
3.	Analog Devices [165]	ADSP 21362 [172]	Floating	32 bits	Single	Not supporting	3MB SRAM, 4MB ROM	333MHz
4.	Analog Devices [165]	ADSP 21261 [173]	Floating	32 bits	Single	Not supporting	1MB SRAM, 3MB ROM	200MHz
5.	Texas Instruments [166]	TMS320C 5515 [174]	Fixed	32 bits	Single	Not supporting	320K RAM, 128K ROM, 4MB SDRAM	120MHz
6.	Texas Instruments [166]	TMS320C 5505 [175]	Fixed	32 bits	Single	Not supporting	320K RAM, 128K ROM,	100MHz
7.	Texas Instruments [166]	TMS320C 6713 [119]	Floating	32 bits	Single	Supporting	16MB SDRAM, 512KB Flash ROM	225MHz
8.	Texas Instruments [166]	TMS320C 6711 [176]	Floating	32 bits	Single	Supporting	16MB SDRAM, 128KB Flash ROM	200MHz
9.	Free-scale Semiconductors [167]	MSC8151 [177]	Floating	32 bits	Single	Not supporting	512 KB L2 cache 32 KB I-cache, 32KB D-cache	1000MHz
10.	Free-scale Semiconductors [167]	MSC8251 [178]	Floating	32 bits	Single	Not supporting	512 KB L2 cache 32 KB I-cache, 32KB D-cache, 1MB RAM	1000MHz
11.	Hyperstone [168]	E1-32XSR [179]	Floating	32 bits	Single	Not supporting	16 KB RAM	220MHz
12.	VeriSilicon [169]	ZSP 400 [180]	Fixed	16 bits	Single	Not supporting	1MB	200MHz

The following characteristics of DSPs are chosen to narrow down the choice [118].

1. Fixed point or floating point
2. External memory bus (bits)
3. Number of cores
4. VLIF architecture
5. On-chip memory
6. Operating clock frequency

For biomedical applications, a floating-point processor is needed to represent accurate discrete values of signals at particular samples [122], and a large memory is needed to store the large number of signals. Moreover, very long instruction word (VLIW) facility is also an added advantage. Most of the high-performance processors have depended on Instruction Level Parallelism (ILP) to achieve high execution speed. ILP processors achieve their high performance by causing multiple operations to execute in parallel, using a combination of compiler and hardware techniques. VLIW is one particular style of processor design that tries to achieve high levels of instruction level parallelism by executing long instruction words composed of multiple operations. The long instruction word called a MultiOp consists of multiple arithmetic, logic and control operations each of which would probably be an individual operation on a simple RISC processor. The VLIW processor concurrently executes the set of operations within a MultiOp thereby achieving instruction level parallelism.

Our literature study of various processors revealed that the Texas TMS320C6x family would make the best embedded processor for the real time implementation of ECG adaptive noise canceller. DSPs in this family of processors are fast, special purpose microprocessors with a specialized type of architecture and an instruction set suitable for signal processing. The C6x notation is used to designate a member of Texas Instruments (TI) TMS320C6000 family of DSPs. Based on a very-long-instruction-word

(VLIW) architecture, the C6x is considered to be TI's most powerful processor [119, 121].

The TMS320C62x is a 16-bit fixed point processor and the '67x is a floating-point processor, with 32-bit integer support. In C6x family we consider C6711 and C6713. Between these finally we consider C6713 because of higher clock rate and higher on chip memory. The C6713 DSP Starter Kit (DSK) is a low-cost standalone development platform that enables users to evaluate and develop applications for the TI C67xx DSP family. The DSK also serves as a hardware reference design for the TMS320C6713 DSP. Schematics, logic equations and application notes are available to ease hardware development and reduce time to market. Because of these advantages we have chosen TMS320C6713 DSP for the development of ANCs to remove artefacts from ECG signals.

6.1.1. Features of TMS320C6713 DSP

This processor has an evaluation board called TMS320C6713 DSK. The DSK comes with a full complement of on-board devices that suit a wide variety of applications environment. The key features include [119]:

- TI 320C6713 is a 32-bit floating point processor.
- TI 6713 DSK operates at 225 MHz, sampling frequency is 8KHz to 96KHz.
- It is capable of processing signals up to frequencies 46KHz.
- It can generate signals from 0.02Hz to 15KHz
- It has single voltage power supply 5v, internally 5v input is converted into 1.26v and 3.3v using separate voltage regulators.1.26v is for DSP, 3.3v supply is for other chips on the board.
- It has 16 MB SDRAM, 264KB internal memory.
- It has 512Kbytes Flash memory.
- C6713 architecture has CPU, Peripherals and Memory.

- CPU fetches advanced VLIW to supply up to eight 32-bit instructions during every clock cycle.

6.2. Implementation of Adaptive Noise Cancellers Using the TMS320C6713 DSP

In our experiments the TI TMS320C6713 DSP is a key element. The architecture of the TMS320C6713 is well suited to numerically intensive adaptive signal processing algorithms. The internal memory is structured so that a total of eight instructions can be called every cycle. For example, with a clock rate of 225 MHz, the C6713 is capable of calling eight 32-bit instructions every 1/(225 MHz) or 4.44 ns. The C6713 (C671, C6711) belongs to the family of floating-point processors, whereas the C62xx and C64xx belong to the family of the C6x fixed-point processors. The C6713 is also capable of fixed-point processing and it enables the developer to update the algorithm to a fixed-point calculation after running under floating point on the same DSK. A typical block diagram of C6713 is shown in Figure 6.2 [119].

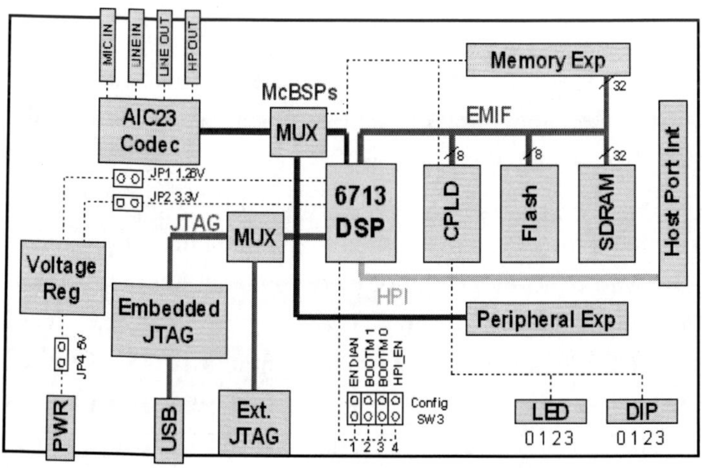

Figure 6.2. Block diagram of TMS320C6713 DSP.

The DSP on the 6713 DSK interfaces to on-board peripherals through a 32-bit wide external memory interface (EMIF). The synchronous RAM (SDRAM), flash and CPLD are all connected to the bus. EMIF signals are also connected daughter card expansion connectors which are used for third party add-in boards. A programmable logic device called a CPLD is used to implement glue logic that ties the board components together. The CPLD has a register-based user interface that lets the user configure the board by reading and writing to its registers. The DSK includes 4 LEDs and a 4 position DIP switch as a simple way to provide the user with interactive feedback. Both are accessed by reading and writing to the CPLD registers. An included 5V external power supply is used to power the board. On-board switching voltage regulators provide the 1.26V DSP core voltage and +3.3V I/O supplies. The board is held in reset until these supplies are within operating specifications. The code composer communicates with the DSK through an embedded Joint Team Action Group (JTAG) emulator with a USB host interface. The DSK can also be used with an external emulator through the external JTAG connector.

In order to facilitate the implementation of the algorithms on the TMS320C6713 MATLAB and C were used. This allowed for rapid development of the ANCs, as well as easy TMS320C6713 assembly code generation and performance monitoring. The embedded target for TI C6713 DSPs and the link for the Code Composer Studio (CCS) toolbox integrate C programs with Texas Instruments DSP tools and allows for the design, simulation, and implementation of signal processing algorithms using blocks from available C libraries.

Figure 6.3 shows the development of a filtering algorithm from the MATLAB model through translation into C and hence to the digital signal processor. For the development of algorithms in the DSK system, the Texas Instrument DSK is provided with an integrated development environment (IDE), called Code Composer Studio (CCS). CCS is a high-level language, with built-in FFT, Wavelet, and other functions for signal processing applications. We can also develop our own functions in C for dedicated and novel applications. The TMS320C6713 DSK has a built in CODEC with a 16-bit register to acquire the ECG signal directly and display it before processing. Only 2048 samples can be viewed at a time but the data can be updated in a circular fashion (the first memory location in the circular memory is moved to the next location and the last memory location is refreshed with the new data). The C code is then linked and transferred to the CCS by the Link for Code Composer Studio. The code is then linked, compiled and loaded to the target by the CCS and finally the DSK processes the signal with the algorithm. The DSK can process up to 5000 samples at a time, but the video buffer can store and view only 2048 samples and circular memory technique is used again to enable sequential display of the processed data.

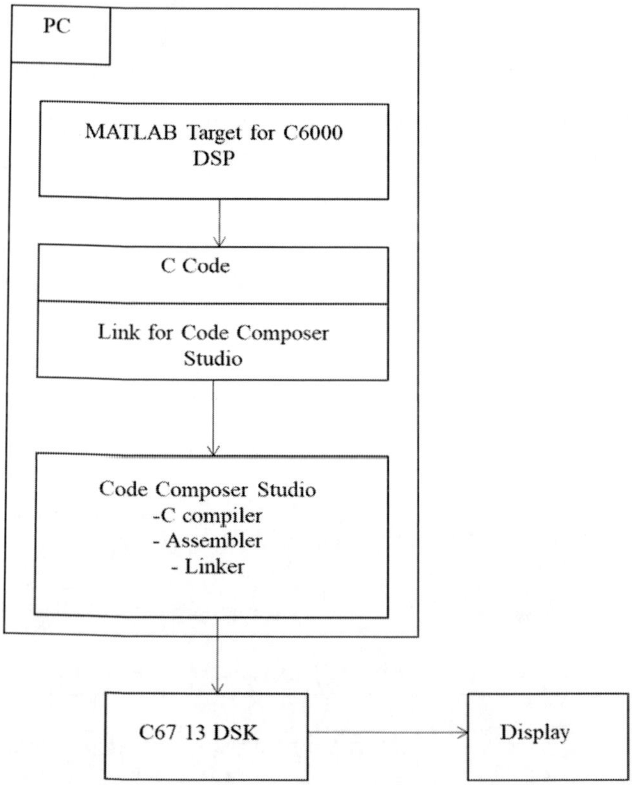

Figure 6.3. Flow diagram of implementation on the DSP.

6.2.1. Procedure for Writing Code Using CCS on the Embedded Processor

Texas Instruments Code Composer Studio (CCS) software is used to develop and test the adaptive noise cancellers on the embedded platform C6713DSK. CCS provides an integrated development environment (IDE) to incorporate the software tools, which include code generation, a C compiler, an assembler, and a linker. It has graphical capabilities, supports real time debugging and is easy to use [118].

Real time analysis can be performed using the real time data exchange (RTDX) associated with the DSP. RTDX allows for data exchange between the host and the target and analysis in real time without stopping the target. The performance of the ANC can be monitored in real time. Through the JTAG communication with on-chip emulation support occurs to control and monitor program execution [187]-[189]. The step by step procedure for the experiment conducted on DSP is illustrated in Figure 6.4 to Figure 6.17.

- Step 1: Choose Open Code Composer Studio with C6713DSK as the target platform.

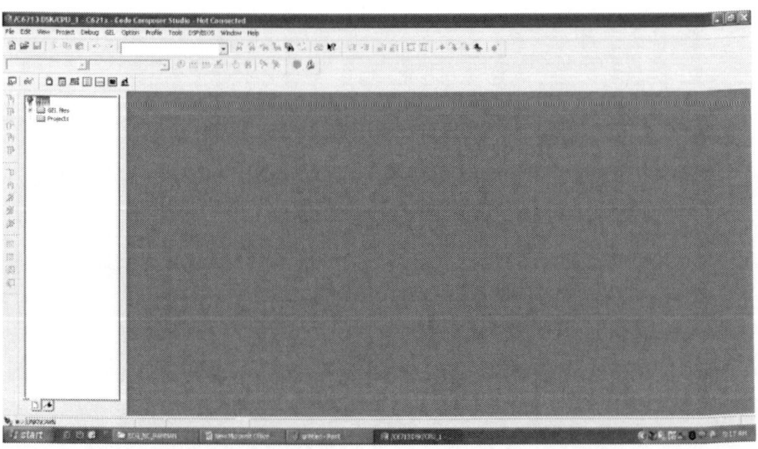

Figure 6.4. Code Composer Studio Window.

- Step 2: Choose to connect the board.

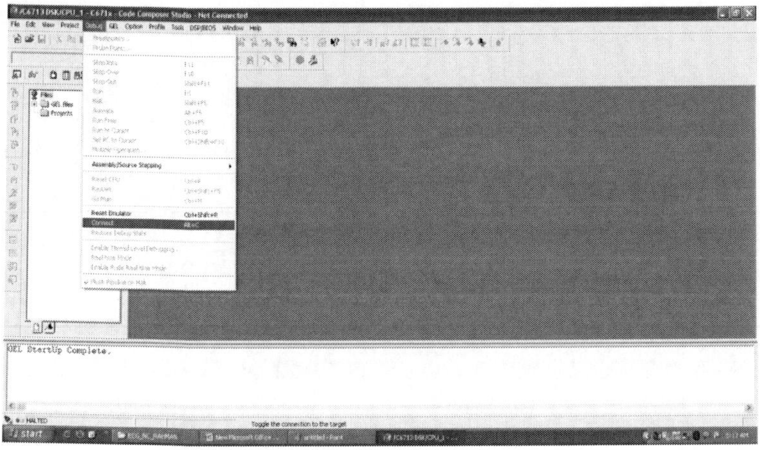

Figure 6.5. DSK 6713 is connected to the project.

- Step 3: Create a new project.

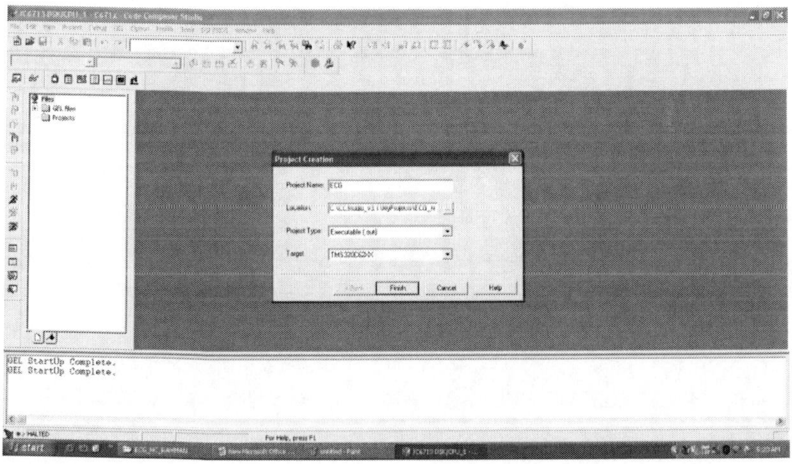

Figure 6.6. A new project is created on DSP.

- Step 4: Choose to create a DSP **BIOS Configuration** file.

File->new->DSP BIOS Configuration File

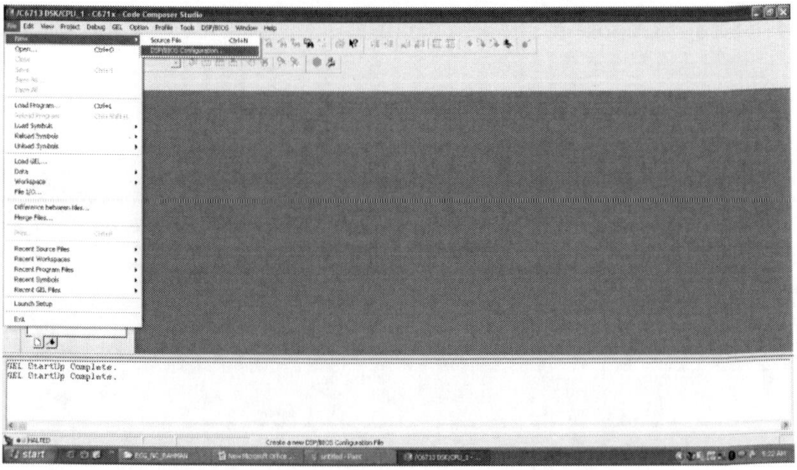

Figure 6.7. DSP BIOS configuration is created.

- Step 5: Choose **dsk6713.cdb** and open the file.

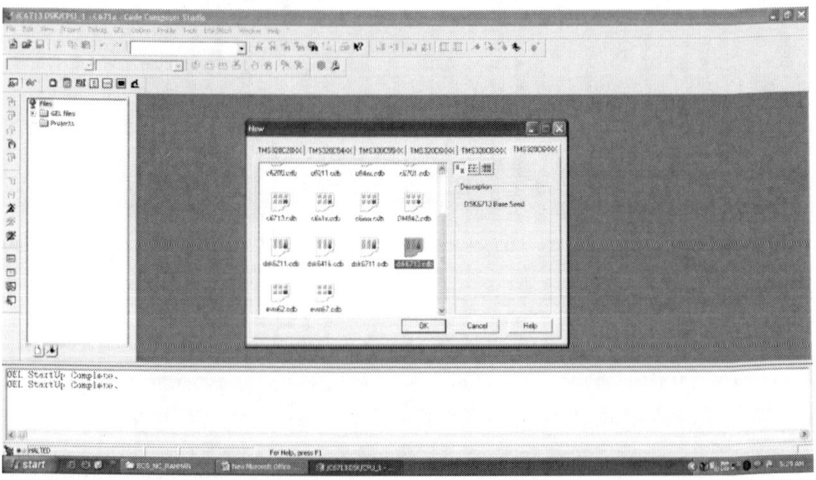

Figure 6.8. Open the dsk6713.cdb file.

- Step 6: Save the Configuration file in the project folder as 'ecg.cdb'.

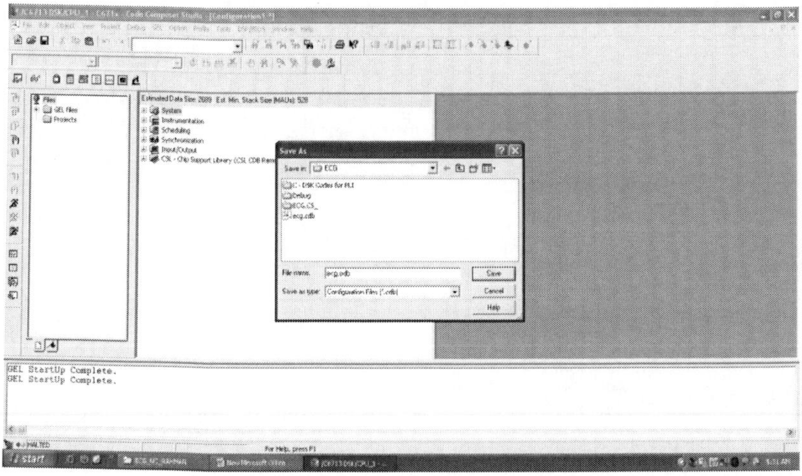

Figure 6.9. The configuration file is stored in the project folder.

- Step 7: Add the Configuration file (ecg.cdb), Source files (C files) and Board Specific Library file (dsk6713dsk.lib).

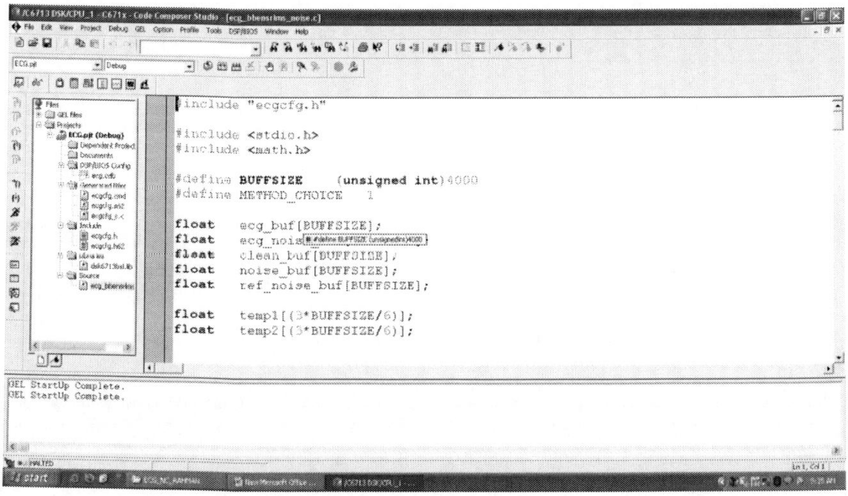

Figure 6.10. Adding .cdb file, source files and library files.

- Step 8: Build the project by choosing Rebuild All.

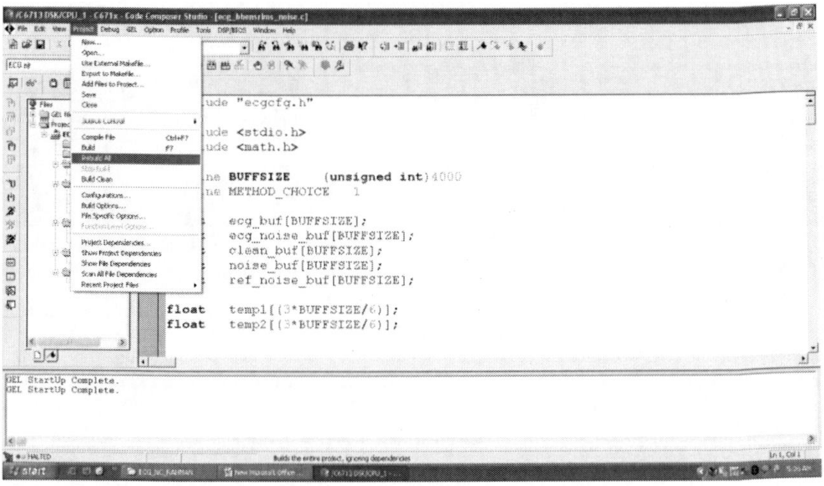

Figure 6.11. Building the project.

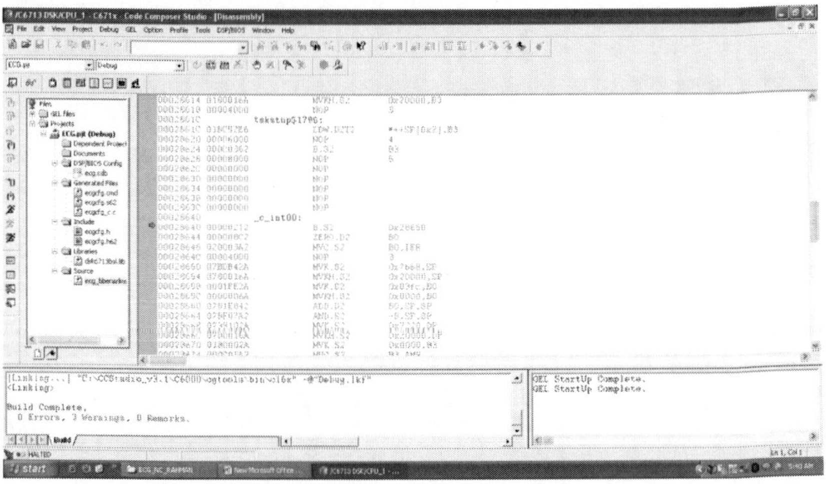

Figure 6.12. Displaying '0 Errors' after building the project.

- Step 9: After successful build of the project, load the data to the buffers in the implementation.

File->Data->Load

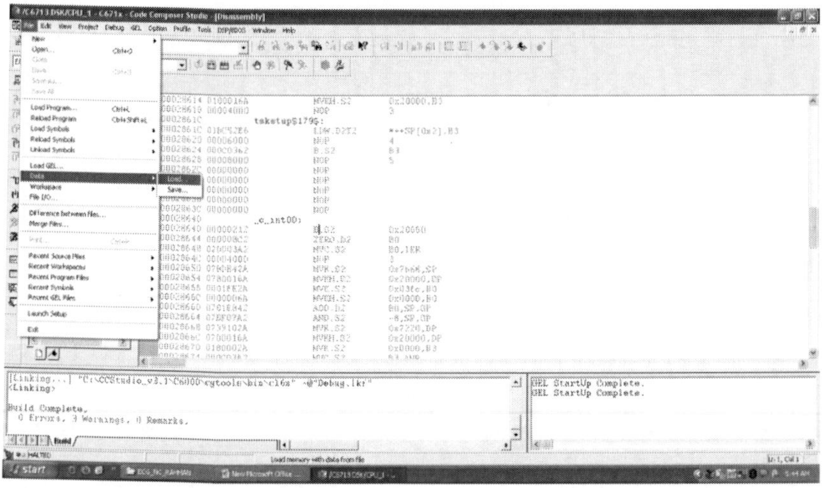

Figure 6.13. Loading data to the buffers.

While loading the data choose 'files of type' as float(.dat).

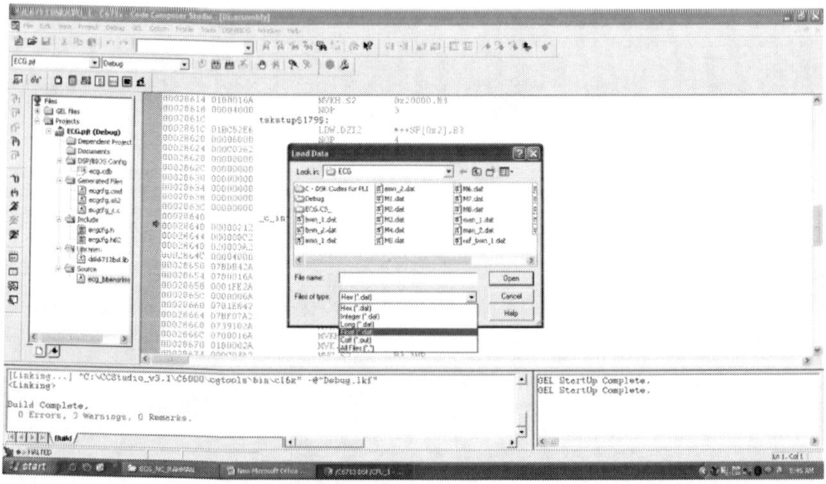

Figure 6.14. Choosing 'files of type' as float.

- Step 10: Run the project.

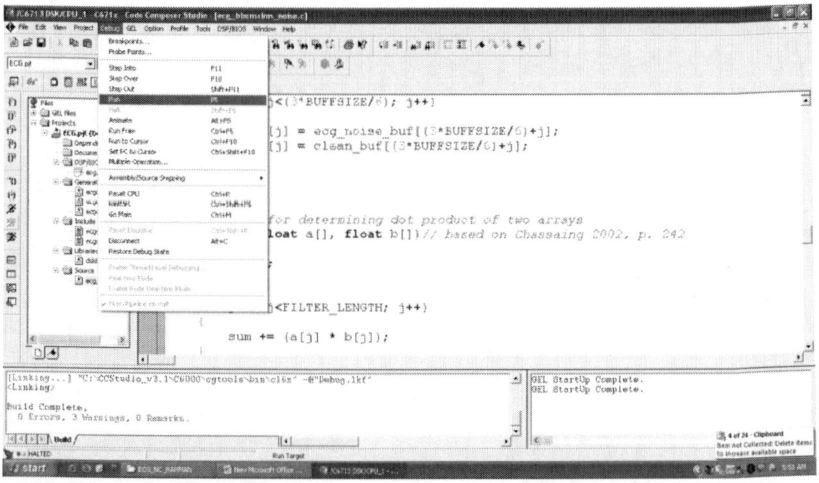

Figure 6.15. Running the project.

- Step 11: Halt the project by setting up Break Point at 'while (1)' loop at the end of 'main' function in the C code.

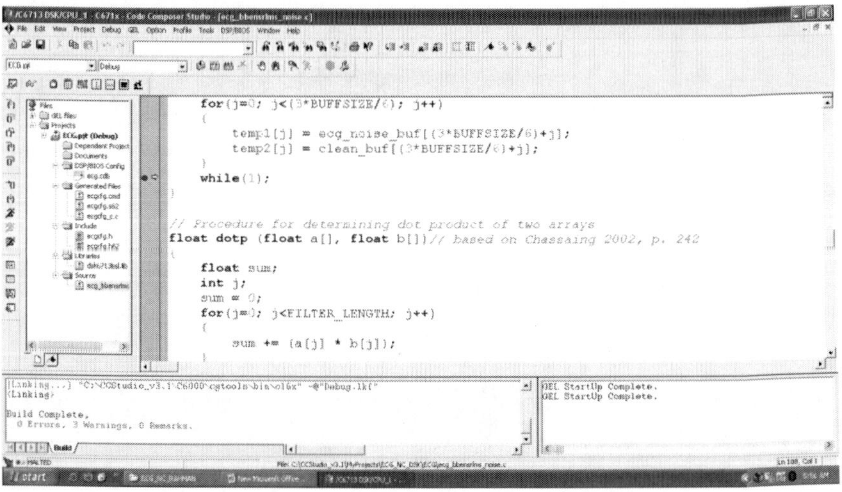

Figure 6.16. Halt the project.

- Step 12: Save the processed data into float type data file.

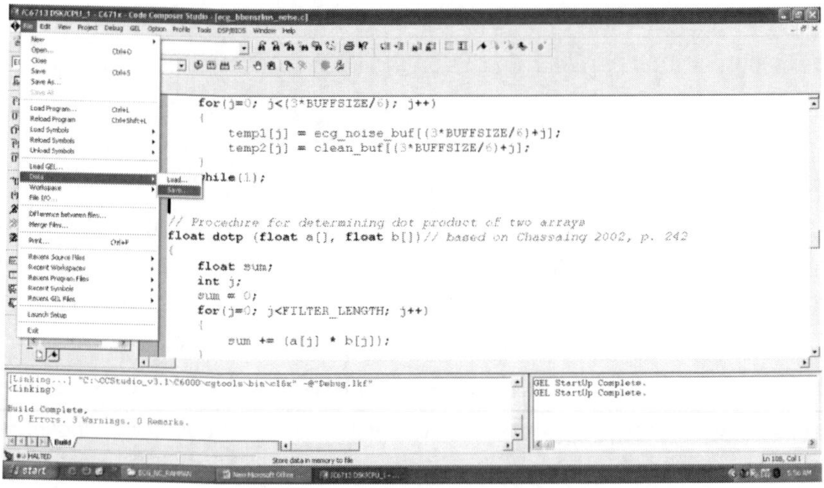

Figure 6.17. Saving the processed data.

The saved data can be displayed using the graphical view of CCS. In this real time implementation, we have chosen LMS, SRLMS and SRDZLMS from Chapter 3, where these algorithms are found to be performed better in simulation studies. Similarly, NSRLMS, ENSRLMS are taken from Chapter 4 and FBNLMS, FBENLMS, BBNSRLMS, BBENSRLMS are taken from Chapter 5. All these algorithms are programmed in C and linked to DSK using CCS. Using these algorithms various ANC structures are implemented on DSP as shown in Figure 2.3.

6.3. Experimental Results and Discussions

For this real-time implementation, we have chosen LMS, SRLMS and SRDZLMS from Chapter 3, as these algorithms performed better in simulation studies. For the same reason, we chose NSRLMS and ENSRLMS from Chapter 4 and FBNLMS, FBENLMS, BBNSRLMS and BBENSRLMS from Chapter 5. All these algorithms are programmed in C and linked to DSK using CCS. We followed the same procedure for the conventional LMS algorithm so that we could use it a benchmark against which to compare the eight chosen algorithms, which were all used to implement various ANC structures on the DSP, as shown in Figure 2.3.

The noisy ECG signal and the reference signal are given as inputs to the DSP, and the required parameters, including step size, variance, filter and block length, taken from the respective MATLAB implementations described in earlier chapters. We considered four of the most important artefacts, Power Line Interference (PLI), Baseline Wander (BW), Muscle Artefacts (MA) and Electrode Motion artefacts (EM). To evaluate the performance, the Signal to Noise Ratio Improvement (SNRI) is measured and compared with that of the conventional LMS algorithm. In the graphs of the results, the x-axis represents the sample number and they-axis represents the amplitude of the signal (note that CCS displays only 2048 samples of a typical ECG). A photograph of the implementation on the TI TMS320C6713 DSP is shown in Figure 6.18. All experiments are performed for 10 times and average values are tabulated.

6.3.1. Adaptive Power-Line Interference Cancellation

This experiment demonstrates PLI cancellation using C6713 DSK. The input to the filter is an ECG signal corrupted with a PLI of amplitude 1mv, frequency 60Hz and sampled at 200Hz. The reference signal is synthesized sinusoidal noise from a noise generator and the output of the filter is the recovered signal. The developed ANCs have the structure shown in Figure 2.3. The contaminated ECG signal is input to DSP $x(n) = s_1 + n_1$, the correlated noise reference is applied as n_2 and the C6713 DSK output is y(n). Various filter structures are implemented using LMS, SRLMS, SRDZLMS, NSRLMS, ENSRLMS, FBNLMS, FBENLMS, BBNSRLMS and BBENSRLMS algorithms. The experimental results using C6713 DSK are shown in Figure 6.19 to Figure 6.27. Two DSP channels are shown. The upper subplot is noisy ECG and the lower the filtered signal obtained with the respective algorithm implemented on the C6713 DSK processor. We have measured the SNRIs for these implementations using (3.25) for ten times and average; these are tabulated in Table 6.2 and compared with MATLAB simulation results.

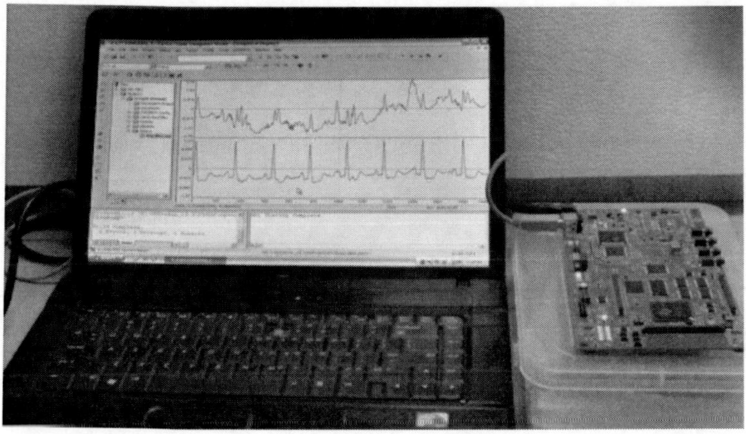

Figure 6.18. Photograph of the implementation on TI TMS320C6713 DSP for removal of EM noise.

The implementation procedure is summarized as follows:

1. Open Code Composer Studio with C6713DSK as the target plot form.
2. Choose to connect the board.
3. Create a new project.
4. Choose to create a DSP BIOS configuration file.
5. Choose DSK6713.cdb and open the file.
6. Save the configuration file in the project folder as ecg.cdb.
7. Add the configuration file (ecg.cdb), source files and board specific library file (dsk6713.lib).
8. Open the project.
9. Choose the adaptive noise canceller developed.
10. Add the source code to the project.
11. Open the C code from source data base.
12. Build the project.

13. After successful build of the project, load the data to the buffers used in the ANC, while loading the data choose file of type as float (.dat).
14. Run the project.
15. Display the noisy signal and filtered signal.

The similar procedure is followed for the remaining noises like BW, MA and EM artefacts.

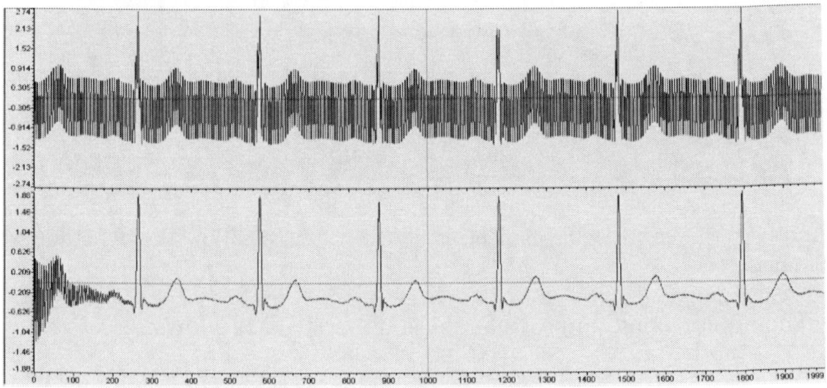

Figure 6.19. Typical filtering results for PLI cancellation using LMS algorithm on DSP.

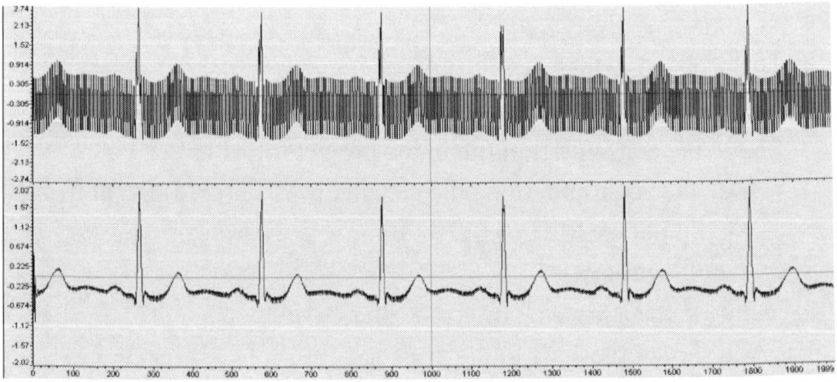

Figure 6.20. Typical filtering results for PLI cancellation using SRLMS algorithm on DSP.

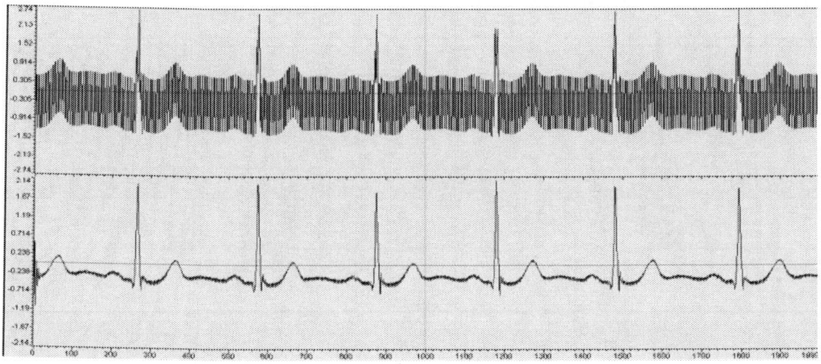

Figure 6.21. Typical filtering results for PLI cancellation using SRDZLMS algorithm on DSP.

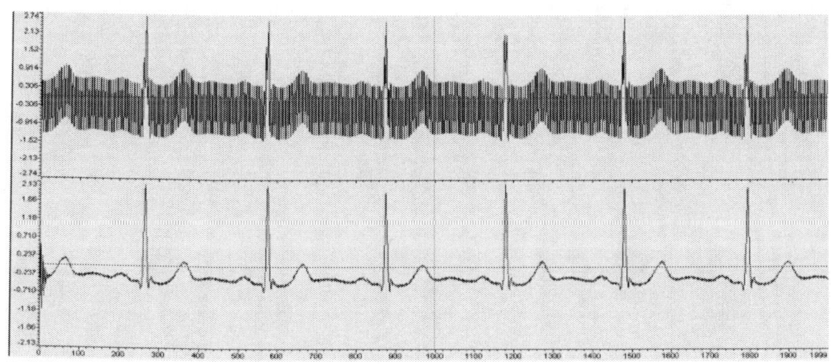

Figure 6.22. Typical filtering results for PLI cancellation using NSRLMS algorithm on DSP.

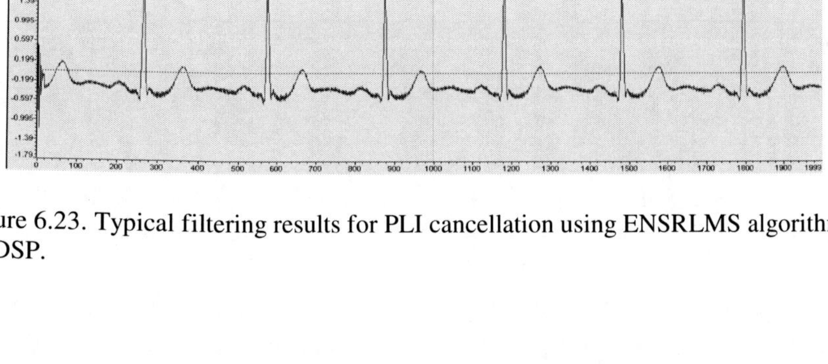

Figure 6.23. Typical filtering results for PLI cancellation using ENSRLMS algorithm on DSP.

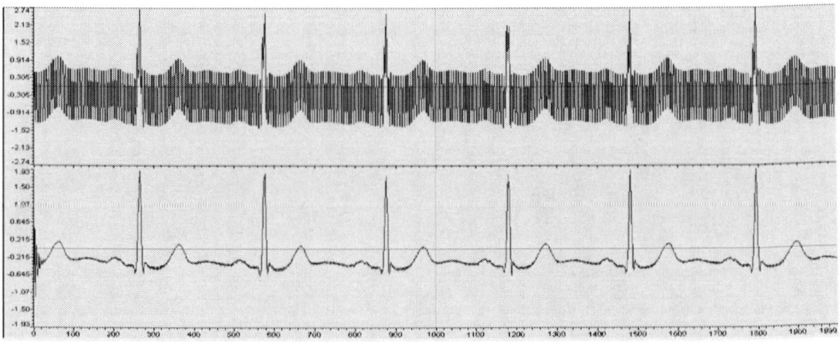

Figure 6.24. Typical filtering results for PLI cancellation using BBNSRLMS algorithm on DSP.

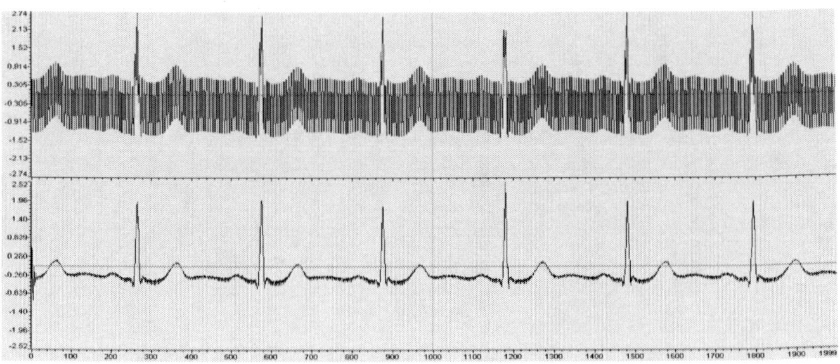

Figure 6.25. Typical filtering results for PLI cancellation using BBENSRLMS algorithm on DSP.

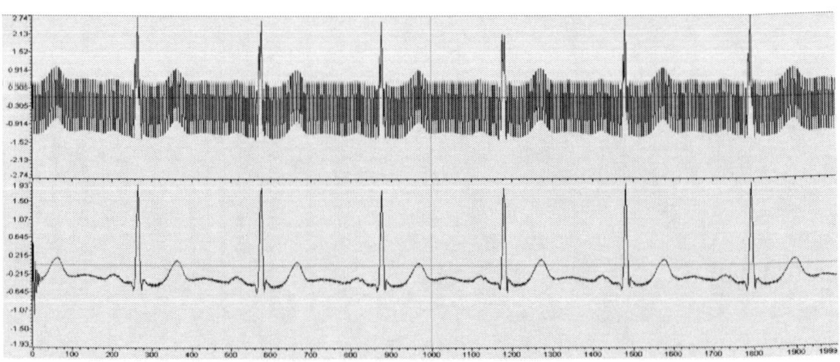

Figure 6.26. Typical filtering results for PLI cancellation using FBNLMS algorithm on DSP.

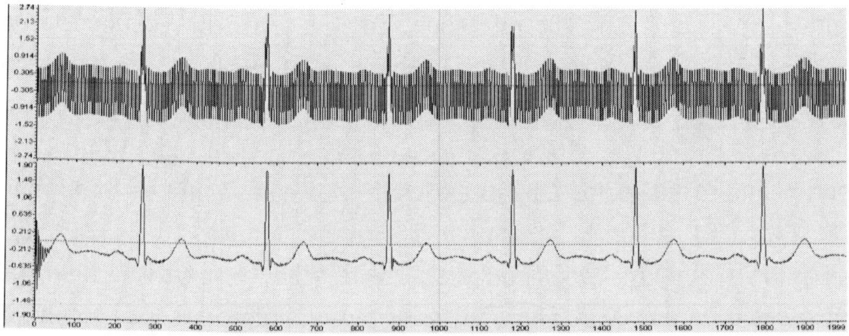

Figure 6.27. Typical filtering results for PLI cancellation using FBENLMS algorithm on DSP.

Table 6.2. SNRI for PLI removal using C6713 realizations

S. No	Algorithm	SNRI in Simulation	SNRI in DSP
1.	LMS	7.2741	6.8760
2.	SRLMS	6.9250	6.4814
3.	DZSRLMS	6.4173	6.0286
4.	NSRLMS	10.8815	10.4281
5.	ENSRLMS	9.5042	9.1257
6.	BBNSRLMS	10.0526	9.7843
7.	BBENSRLMS	10.6998	10.2584
8.	FBNLMS	18.8638	18.3027
9.	FBENLMS	21.0837	20.5203

Table 6.2 clearly shows that the SNRI achieved in processor implementation is closely correlated with the MATLAB simulations. Among the nine ANCs developed, FBENLMS filters PLI efficiently, while SRLMS and DZSRLMS achieves an SNRI very close to that of the LMS, with a single multiplication operation.

6.3.2. Adaptive Baseline Wander Removal

This experiment demonstrates BW cancellation, which is a non-stationary noise cancellation. The input to the filter is an ECG signal contaminated with respiration wander; this is applied to a noise canceller as shown in Figure 2.3. The reference signal is a real BW obtained from the MIT-BIH Noise Stress Test Database. Various filter structures are implemented using LMS, SRLMS, SRDZLMS, NSRLMS, ENSRLMS, FBNLMS, FBENLMS, BBNSRLMS and BBENSRLMS algorithms. The experimental results using C6713 DSK are shown in Figure 6.28 to Figure 6. 36. Two DSP channels are shown. The upper subplot is the noisy ECG, lower the filtered signal obtained with the respective algorithm implemented on the DSP. The SNRIs for these implementations compared with the MATLAB simulation results, are shown in Table 6.3.

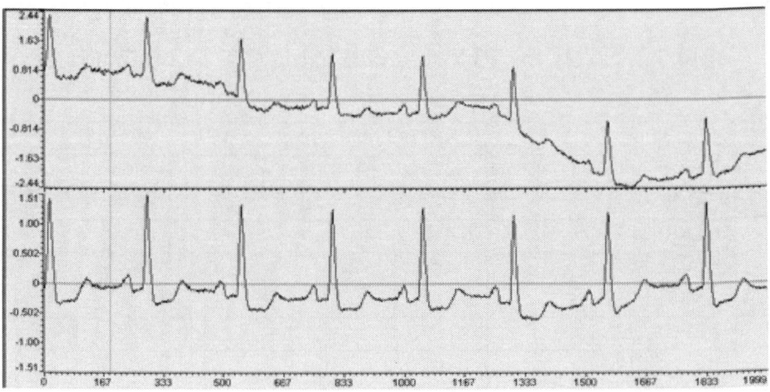

Figure 6.28. Typical filtering results for BW cancellation using LMS algorithm on DSP.

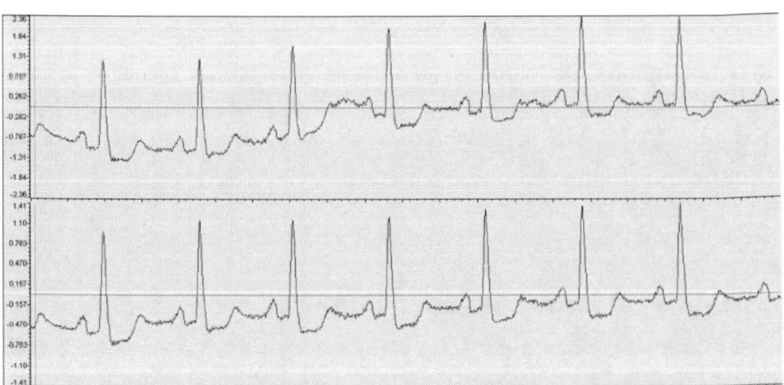

Figure 6.29. Typical filtering results for BW cancellation using SRLMS algorithm on DSP.

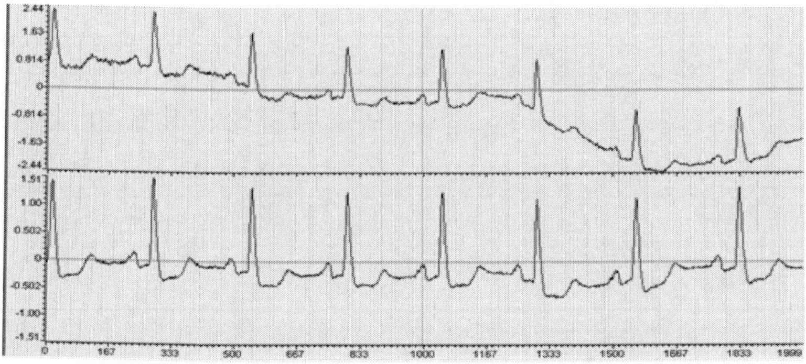

Figure 6.30. Typical filtering results for BW cancellation using DZSRLMS algorithm on DSP.

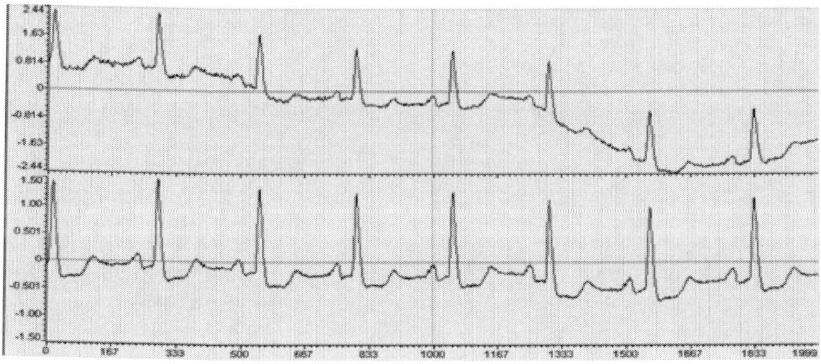

Figure 6.31. Typical filtering results for BW cancellation using NSRLMS algorithm on DSP.

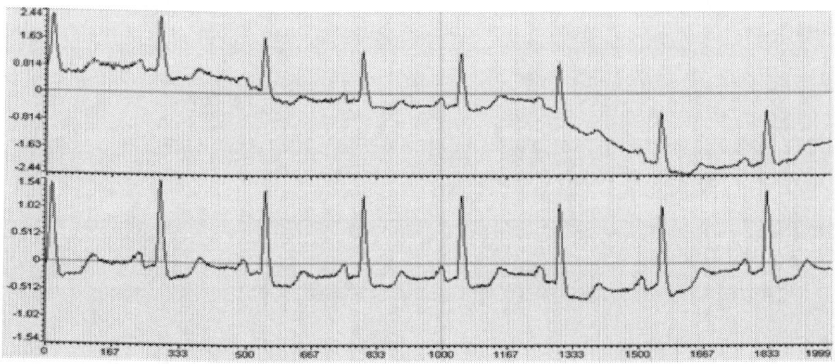

Figure 6.32. Typical filtering results for BW cancellation using ENSRLMS algorithm on DSP.

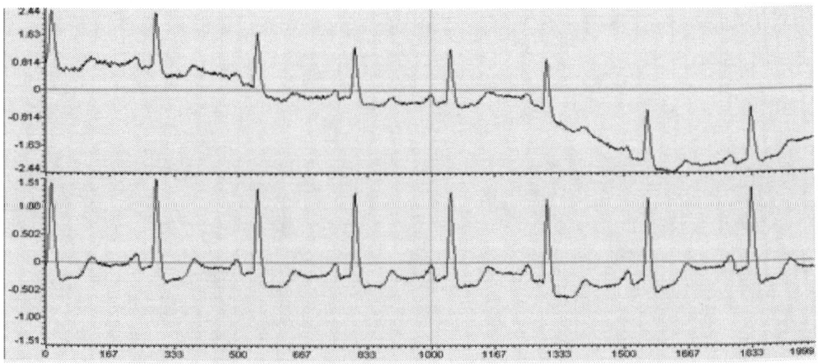

Figure 6.33. Typical filtering results for BW cancellation using BBNSRLMS algorithm on DSP.

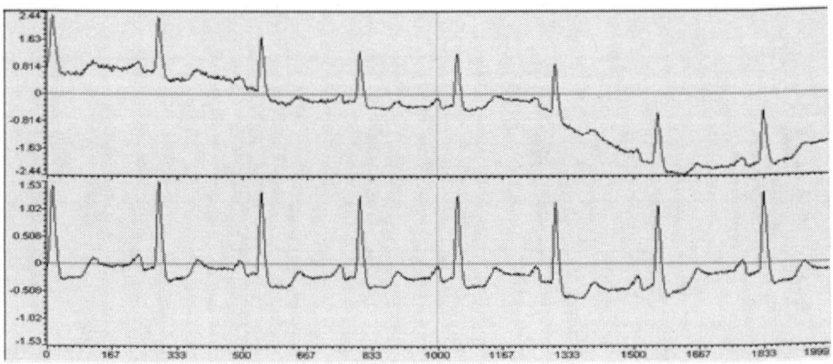

Figure 6.34. Typical filtering results for BW cancellation using BBENSRLMS algorithm on DSP.

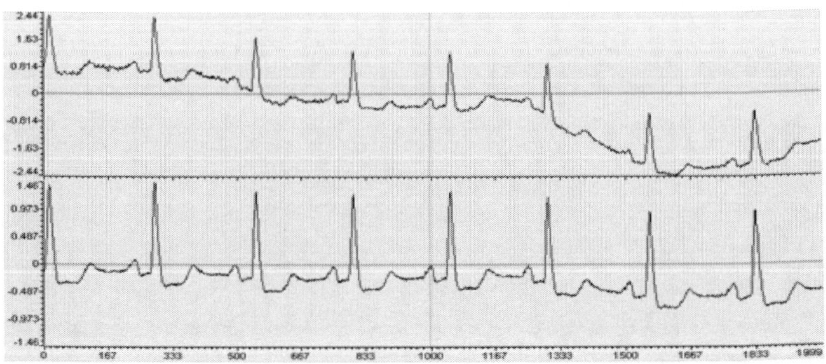

Figure 6.35. Typical filtering results for BW cancellation using FBNLMS algorithm on DSP.

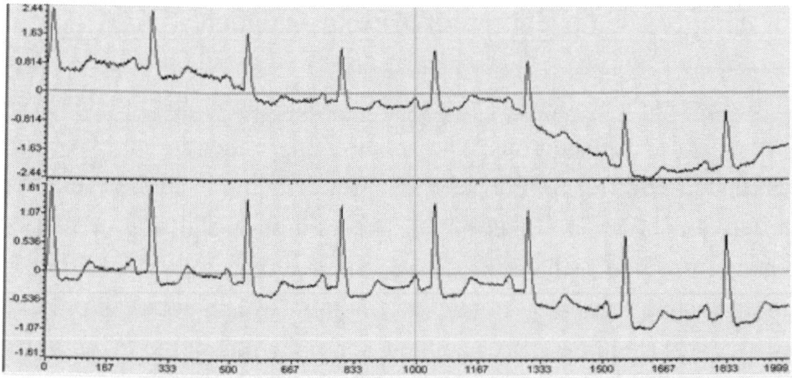

Figure 6.36. Typical filtering results for BW cancellation using FBENLMS algorithm on DSP.

Table 6.3. SNRI for BW removal using C6713 realizations

S. No	Algorithm	SNRI in Simulation	SNRI in DSP
1.	LMS	3.4080	3.2199
2.	SRLMS	2.5390	2.3068
3.	DZSRLMS	4.5439	4.3015
4.	NSRLMS	11.1317	10.7632
5.	ENSRLMS	9.9608	8.9841
6.	BBNSRLMS	9.3007	8.4590
7.	BBENSRLMS	10.1198	9.7987
8.	FBNLMS	13.5793	12.8672
9.	FBENLMS	14.7234	14.3511

From Table 6.3 it is clear that FBENLMS filtering BW noise efficiently by achieving highest SNRI, next place goes to FBNLMS. NSRLMS based filtering also enhances ECG efficiently with a deviation of approximately 2dB from FBNLMS. Because of applying threshold DZSRLMS requires less computations, in this case single multiplication is sufficient and filters the noisy signal effectively with a SNRI greater than LMS filtering, in which required multiplications are equal to the length of the filter.

6.3.3. Adaptive Cancellation of Muscle Artefacts

This experiment demonstrates MA cancellation, which is a non-stationary noise cancellation. The input to the filter is an ECG signal contaminated with respiration baseline wander; this is applied to a noise canceller, as shown in Figure 2.3. The reference signal is a real MA obtained from the MIT-BIH Noise Stress Test Database. The MA originally had a sampling frequency of 360 Hz and were anti-alias re-sampled to 128Hz in order to match the sampling rate of the ECG. Various filter structures are implemented using LMS, SRLMS, SRDZLMS, NSRLMS, ENSRLMS, FBNLMS, FBENLMS, BBNSRLMS and BBENSRLMS algorithms. We have displayed two channels of the DSP. The upper subplot is noisy ECG and the lower subplot is filtered signal using respective algorithm implemented on C6713 DSK processor. The experimental results using C6713 DSK are shown in Figure 6.37 to Figure 6. 45. The SNRI for these realizations are shown in Table 6.4, compared with MATLAB simulation results.

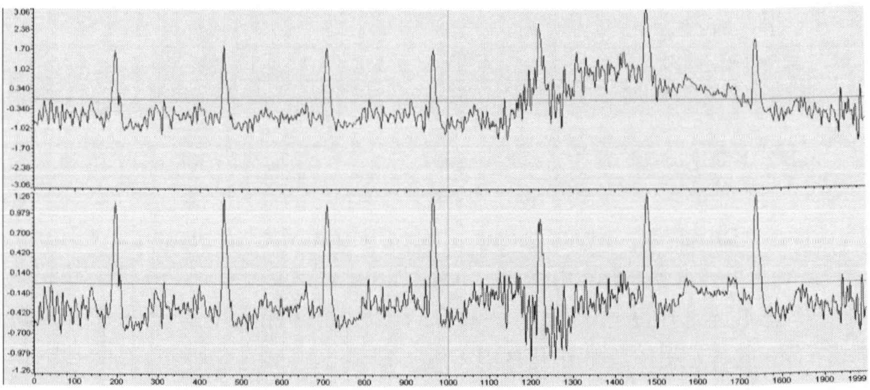

Figure 6.37. Typical filtering results for MA cancellation using LMS algorithm on DSP.

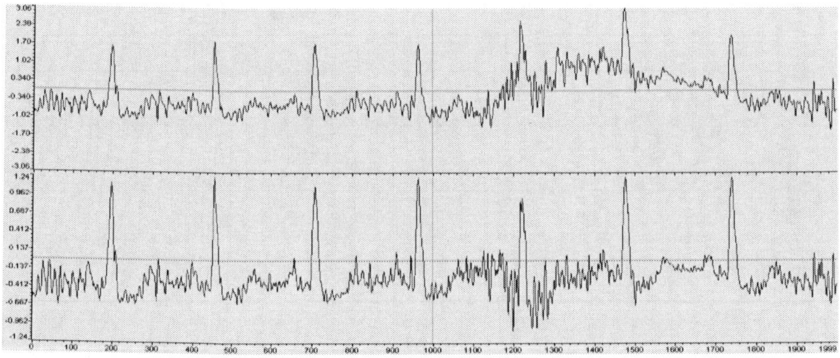

Figure 6.38. Typical filtering results for MA cancellation using SRLMS algorithm on DSP.

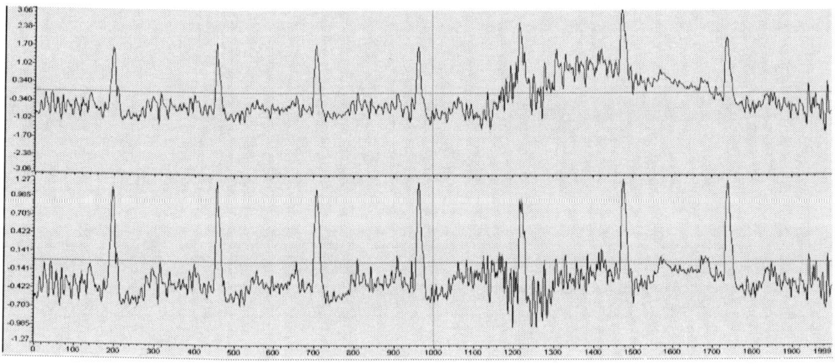

Figure 6.39. Typical filtering results for MA cancellation using DZSRLMS algorithm on DSP.

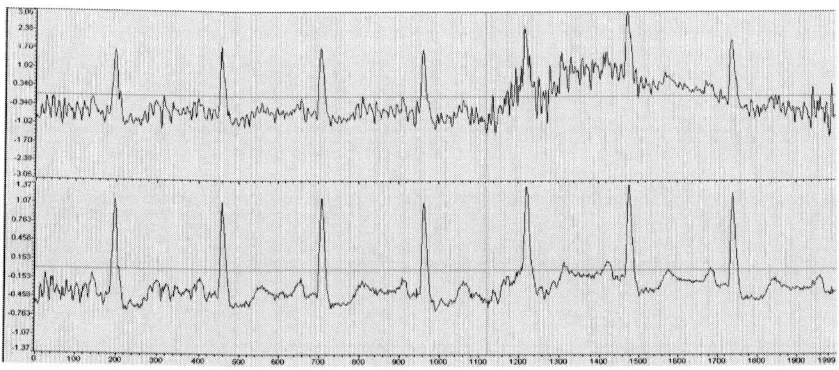

Figure 6.40. Typical filtering results for MA cancellation using NSRLMS algorithm on DSP.

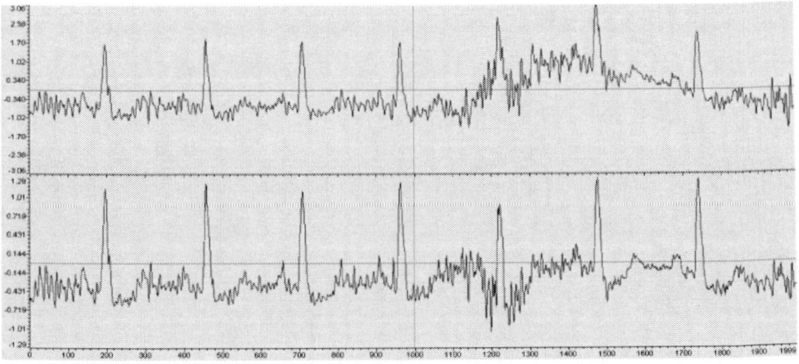

Figure 6.41. Typical filtering results for MA cancellation using ENSRLMS algorithm on DSP.

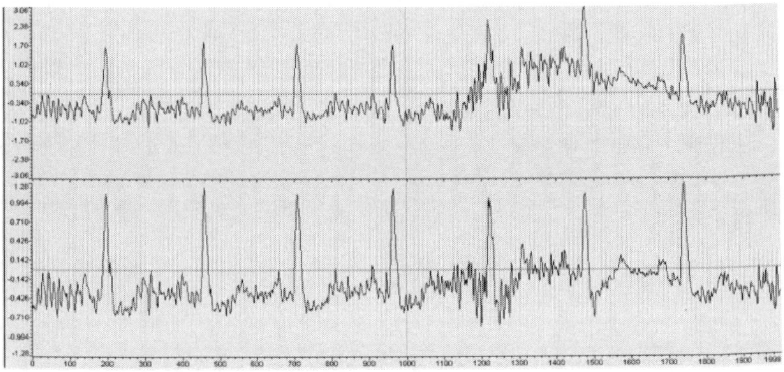

Figure 6.42. Typical filtering results for MA cancellation using BBNSRLMS algorithm on DSP.

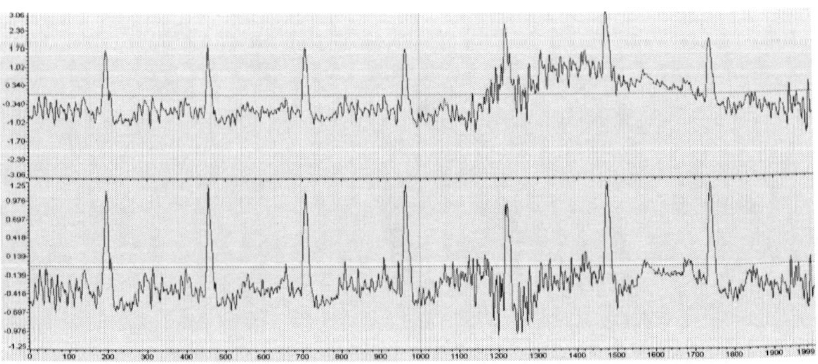

Figure 6.43. Typical filtering results for MA cancellation using BBENSRLMS algorithm on DSP.

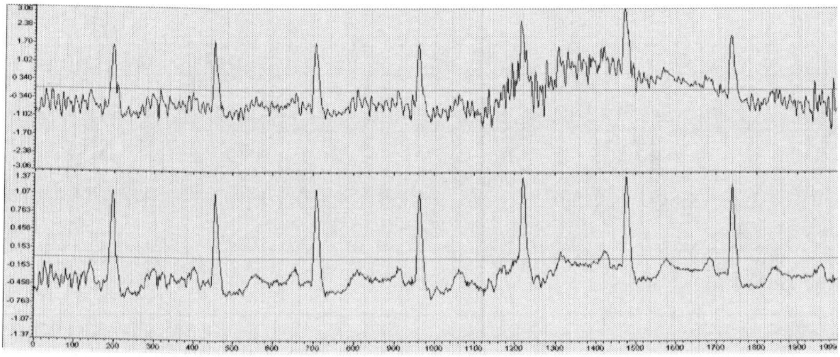

Figure 6.44. Typical filtering results for MA cancellation using FBNLMS algorithm on DSP.

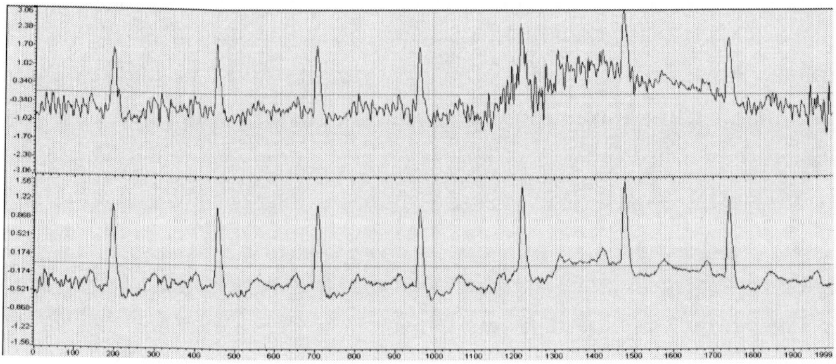

Figure 6.45. Typical filtering results for MA cancellation using FBENLMS algorithm on DSP.

Table 6.4. SNRI for MA removal using C6713 realizations

S. No	Algorithm	SNRI in Simulation	SNRI in DSP
1.	LMS	4.6154	4.3807
2.	SRLMS	3.5043	3.2364
3.	DZSRLMS	4.8520	4.4197
4.	NSRLMS	10.3672	9.9750
5.	ENSRLMS	9.5483	9.0421
6.	BBNSRLMS	8.6025	8.1637
7.	BBENSRLMS	10.1530	9.7591
8.	FBNLMS	15.9532	14.1786
9.	FBENLMS	16.0748	15.2355

The SNRI measurements for adaptive MA removal are shown in Table 6.4, for consistency of the results we made 10 SNRI measurements and took the average. From the table it is clear that frequency domain filtering increases the resolution of the signal by achieving a high SNRI. The normalization-based algorithms all perform approximately uniformly, and the DZSRLMS with single multiplication achieves SNRI greater than that of the LMS based ANC.

6.3.4. Adaptive Cancellation of Electrode Motion Artefacts

This experiment demonstrates EM cancellation, which is a non-stationary noise cancellation. The input to the filter is ECG signal is contaminated with respiration baseline wander; this is applied to a noise canceller shown in Figure 2.3. The reference signal is a real EM obtained from MIT-BIH Noise Stress Test Database. The EM originally had a sampling frequency of 360Hz and therefore they were anti-alias re-sampled to 128Hz in order to match the sampling rate of the ECG. Various filter structures are implemented using LMS, SRLMS, SRDZLMS, NSRLMS, ENSRLMS, FBNLMS, FBENLMS, BBNSRLMS and BBENSRLMS algorithms. We have displayed two channels of the DSP. The upper subplot is noisy ECG and the lower subplot is filtered signal using respective algorithm implemented on C6713 DSK processor. The experimental results using C6713 DSK are shown in Figure 6.46 to Figure 6. 54. The SNRI for these realizations are shown in Table 6.5, compared with MATLAB simulation results.

Table 6.5 confirms the close correlation between the simulation and experimental results. All the algorithms successfully filter artefacts from ECG signals. FBENLMS and FBNLMS perform better than the others, and of the normalization algorithms NSRLMS achieves the best SNRI with less than 1dB deviation from FBNLMS. For these artefacts DZSRLMS achieves a better SNRI than the LMS algorithm does.

Table 6.5. SNRI for EM removal using C6713 realizations

S. No	Algorithm	SNRI in Simulation	SNRI in DSP
1.	LMS	3.9484	3.6172
2.	SRLMS	2.8020	2.3165
3.	DZSRLMS	4.8700	4.2942
4.	NSRLMS	12.2121	11.5380
5.	ENSRLMS	10.2890	9.3927
6.	BBNSRLMS	10.2849	9.3574
7.	BBENSRLMS	11.5198	10.6911
8.	FBNLMS	13.3706	12.4572
9.	FBENLMS	14.5783	13.3190

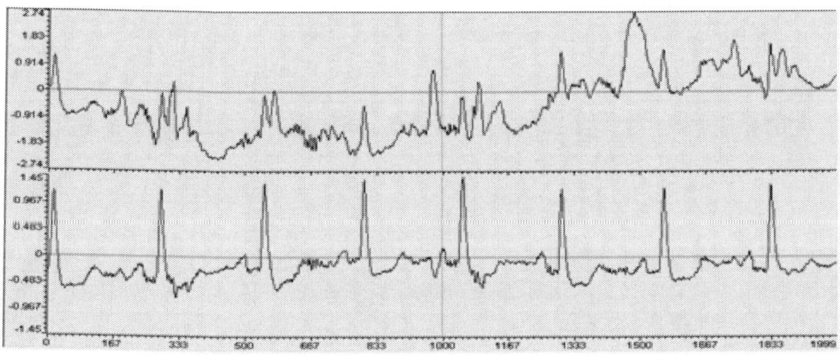

Figure 6.46. Typical filtering results for EM cancellation using LMS algorithm on DSP.

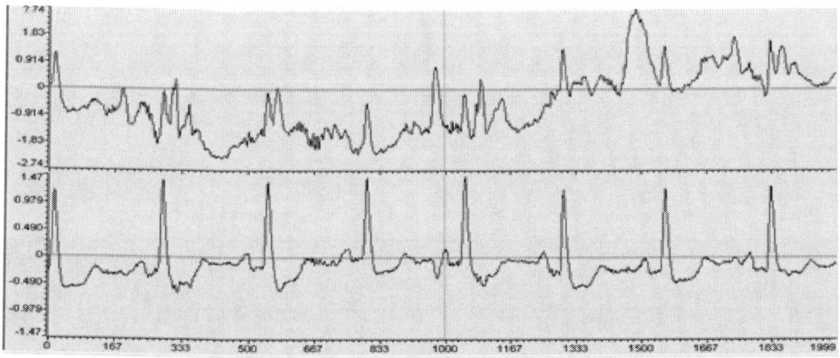

Figure 6.47. Typical filtering results for EM cancellation using SRLMS algorithm on DSP.

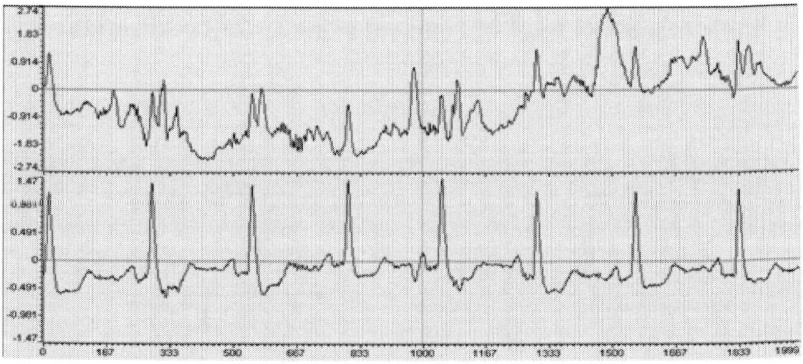

Figure 6.48. Typical filtering results for EM cancellation using SRDZLMS algorithm on DSP.

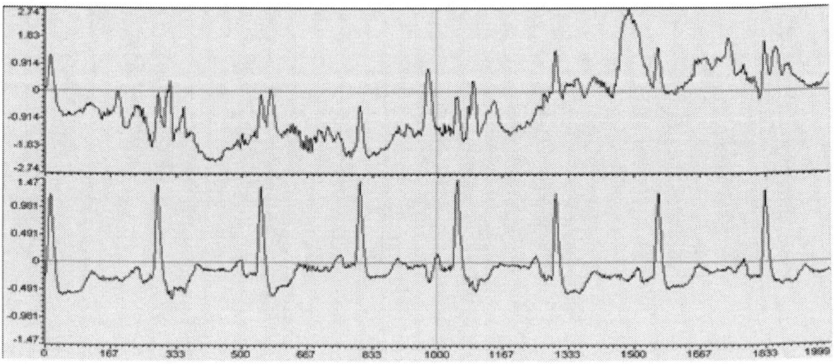

Figure 6.49. Typical filtering results for EM cancellation using NSRLMS algorithm on DSP.

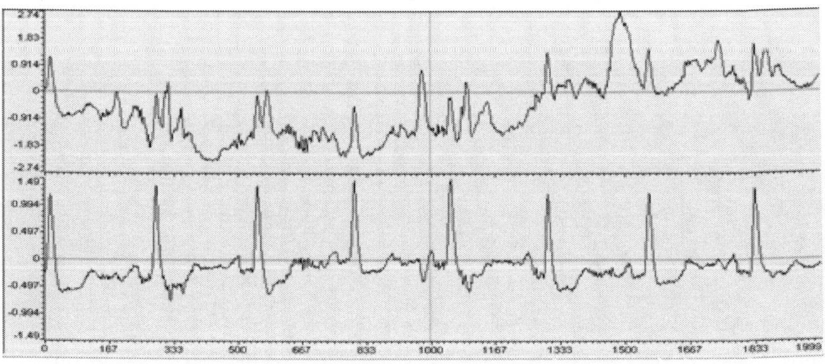

Figure 6.50. Typical filtering results for EM cancellation using ENSRLMS algorithm on DSP.

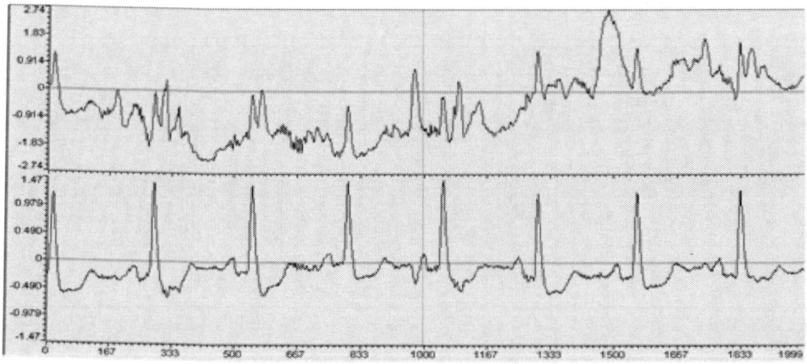

Figure 6.51. Typical filtering results for EM cancellation using BBNSRLMS algorithm on DSP.

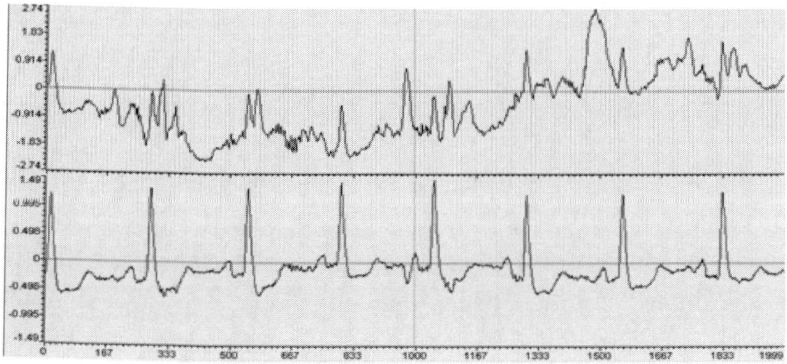

Figure 6.52. Typical filtering results for EM cancellation using BBENSRLMS algorithm on DSP.

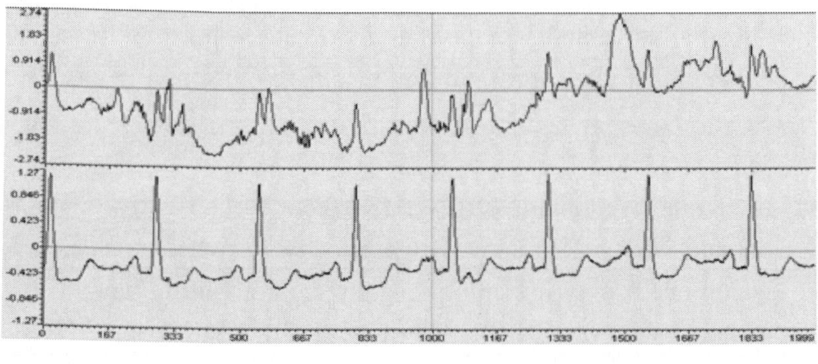

Figure 6.53. Typical filtering results for EM cancellation using FBNLMS algorithm on DSP.

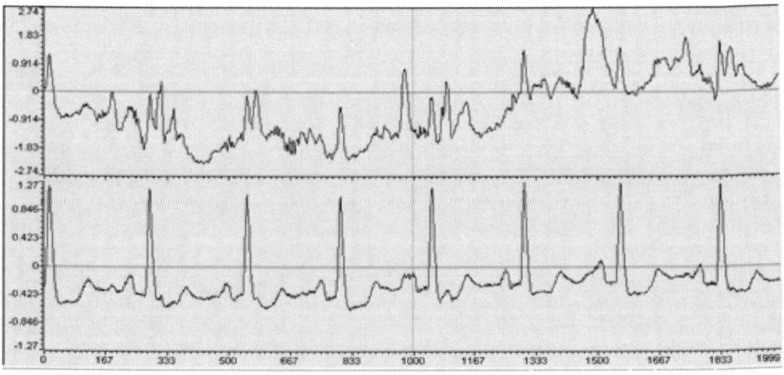

Figure 6.54. Typical filtering results for EM cancellation using FBENLMS algorithm on DSP.

6.4. Conclusion

Of the eight ANCs used in real time implementations on embedded DSP FBNLMS and FBENLMS achieved higher SNRIs because they used frequency domain processing. The normalization factor meant that sign-based algorithms performs better than the fixed step size algorithms. Among the normalized algorithms, NSRLMS performance was best with respect to SNRI and convergence, it needs only one multiplication to compute the weight update equation. These are shown in Tables 6.2 - 6.5 for PLI, BW, MA and EM cancellation respectively. The SNRI values obtained in simulation studies are closely correlates with those obtained in the experimental studies. From these results the following points are concluded:

- In frequency domain FBENLMS filters PLI effectively, in time domain NSRLMS removes PLI effectively, whereas SRDZLMS, which needs only one multiplication for computing weight update equation achieves SNRI greater than that of LMS based ANC.
- For the removal of non-stationary noises i.e., BW, MA and EM also the frequency domain FBENLMS, NSRLMS and DZSRLMS algorithms performs efficiently.

These algorithms are therefore suited for telecardiology applications, where high SNR and minimal computations are desirable.

Chapter 7

CONCLUSION

7.1. INTRODUCTION

It is evident from this work that there is a great need of developing the new ANCs for noise cancellation in ECG signals due to PLI, BW, MA, EM and channel noise specially in biotelemetry. Conventional methods using the LMS algorithm are serving the purpose to a little extent. So, to enhance the ability of the ANCs we have done work on developing the new ANCs and succeeded greatly. To prove this, we developed various adaptive noise cancellers, using three categories of adaptive algorithms to achieve fast convergence, high signal to noise ratio and low computational complexity. These are,

1. Weight update variants of LMS algorithm
2. Normalized adaptive algorithms
3. Block adaptive algorithms

In the present work we have developed 42 new ANCs and tested them in simulations using MATLAB. The eight best performing algorithms were then tested on a real time embedded system. All worked much more efficiently than conventional ANCs, and their performance is reviewed in the following sections.

7.2. Review of Sign Based Adaptive Noise Cancellers

In Chapter 3, we considered weight update variants of the LMS algorithm namely Leaky LMS, Dead zone LMS, LMF and Median LMS algorithms and proved that the developed ANCs remove the artefacts in ECG signals efficiently. In the noise canceller, input and desired signals are properly chosen in such that the filter output is the best squared estimate of the original signal. For this we considered four dominant artefacts, power line interference, baseline wander, muscle artefacts and electrode motion artefacts along with random channel noise. To achieve a fast data transmission rate, reduced computational complexity is needed, and this can be accomplished by clipping either the estimation error or the input data. The three versions of signed algorithms SRA, SA and SS make use of this clipping, so we extended the LMS based adaptive algorithms to make them into sign based adaptive algorithms. These were used to develop ANCs that were tested on ECG signals. To evaluate their performance, we measured computational complexity, EMSE, misadjustment, SNRI and convergence characteristics are plotted.

Among the five LMS based algorithms DZLMS and LMF removed non-stationary noise the best. Among the sign-based versions the SRLMS, SRLLMS, DZSRLMS, SRLMF, SRMLMS algorithms gave the best performances with respect to convergence, SNRI, EMSE, misadjustment and computational complexity. All the remaining SA and SSA based ANCs are slightly inferior to their LMS counterpart. The sign-sign version of the LMS based algorithm does not use multiplication, and weight updating can be performed with addition and sign check operations.

From Table 7.1 it is evident that among the algorithms developed to reduce computational complexity and increase SNRI, SRLMS and

SRDZLMS ANCs were selected for implementation on the embedded DSP and compared with standard LMS based ANC.

Table 7.1. Performance comparison of sign algorithms in terms of SNRI (dBs)

S. No.	Algorithm	Average SNRI for PLI Removal	Average SNRI for BW Removal	Average SNRI for MA Removal	Average SNRI for EM Removal
1.	LMS	7.6095	2.7488	4.6128	3.3366
2.	LLMS	8.6110	3.1006	4.7189	3.6065
3.	DZLMS	8.0244	3.9099	5.4386	4.7587
4.	LMF	8.1521	3.9080	5.4617	4.8943
5.	MLMS	8.2756	3.0470	4.5069	3.9536
6.	**SRLMS**	**7.3394**	**2.4080**	**2.9024**	**2.5771**
7.	SLMS	7.0053	2.1121	2.5556	2.3340
8.	SSLMS	6.6647	1.5722	2.2385	2.0515
9.	SRLLMS	8.1497	2.4954	2.5089	2.3672
10.	SLLMS	5.4627	2.1082	1.9371	2.0581
11.	SSLLMS	4.4476	1.7447	1.6065	1.7845
12.	**SRDZLMS**	**7.6283**	**3.8610**	**4.0833**	**4.0097**
13.	SDZLMS	7.3185	2.9783	3.2148	2.5337
14.	SSDZLMS	6.1753	2.4358	2.3420	1.3718
15.	SRLMF	7.5198	3.0612	3.7426	3.8439
16.	SLMF	7.0053	2.1121	2.5556	2.3340
17.	SSLMF	6.6647	1.5722	2.2385	2.0515
18.	SRMLMS	7.4461	2.9125	2.9557	2.4523
19.	SMLMS	6.6330	2.3106	2.6240	2.0565
20	SSMLMS	6.0163	1.9031	2.1909	1.8153

7.3. Review of Normalization Based Adaptive Noise Cancellers

In Chapter 4, the problem of noise cancelation from ECG signal using sign based normalized adaptive filters are proposed and tested on real signals with different artefacts obtained from the MIT-BIH database. For this, the input and the desired response signals are properly chosen in such a way that the filter output is the best least squared estimate of the original

ECG signal. We developed two types of normalized filters, called data normalized and error normalized. These are commonly known as NLMS and ENLMS algorithms respectively. To reduce computational complexity, we successfully developed various ANCs that use sign-based versions of both NLMS and ENLMS. Between NLMS and ENLMS the performance of NLMS is found to be better in terms of SNRI, EMSE and M_{ad}.

From the two normalized algorithm versions we derived and developed six sign-based versions of algorithms with low complexity, making a total of eight algorithms. Of the six sign-based algorithms NSRLMS performed best, followed by ENSRLMS, NSLMS, NSSLMS, ENSLMS and ENSSLMS in that order. All of them had a better filtering performance and lower computational complexity than the LMS algorithm (expect that one division operation is needed for normalization). From the simulation results it is clear that the proposed ANCs remove non-stationary noise efficiently. The proposed treatment provides a high signal to noise ratio and lower computational complexity, making sign-based algorithms are more suitable for wireless biotelemetry ECG systems. A comparison of average SNRI of normalized algorithms is shown in Table 7.2.

Table 7.2. Performance comparison of normalized algorithms in terms of SNRI (dBs)

S. No.	Algorithm	Average SNRI for PLI Removal	Average SNRI for BW Removal	Average SNRI for MA Removal	Average SNRI for EM Removal
1.	NLMS	11.8320	10.1599	10.5634	11.1647
2.	ENLMS	10.4010	9.1807	9.5711	9.9206
3.	**NSRLMS**	**11.7749**	**9.6426**	**9.9381**	**10.6022**
4.	NSLMS	9.2767	8.3125	7.9674	8.2805
5.	NSSLMS	8.1543	6.9880	6.5227	7.4741
6.	**ENSRLMS**	**9.9204**	**9.0121**	**9.0588**	**9.2077**
7.	ENSLMS	7.9942	6.6099	7.7801	7.0363
8.	ENSSLMS	7.1865	5.7252	6.9314	6.0217

Based on computational complexity and SNRI among all the algorithms we have chosen NSRLMS and ENSRLMS based ANCs for implementation in a real time environment on a digital signal processor.

7.4. Review of Block Based Adaptive Noise Cancellers

In Chapter 5, we proposed and developed overlapping, non-overlapping block adaptive filters for noise cancellation in ECG signals. These were tested on real signals, contaminated with different artefacts, obtained from MIT-BIH database. In the noise canceller, input and desired signals are properly chosen such that the filter output is the best squared estimate of the original signal.

First, we developed adaptive filters using the BLMS algorithm. The convergence characteristics of BLMS are approximately similar to that of LMS algorithm. However due to signal averaging reduces the amplitude of the ECG signal, however, leading to low SNR. To improve convergence rate and filtering capability we applied both data-normalization and error-normalization to block adaptive filters, resulting the BNLMS and BENLMS algorithms. Our experiments proved that normalization improves filtering capability. These block algorithms were also implemented in frequency domain viz., FBLMS, FBNLMS and FBENLMS algorithms. Frequency domain treatment improves the resolution and SNR.

Based on computational complexity and SNRI among all the algorithms we have chosen FBNLMS and FBENLMS based ANCs for implementation in real time environment on a digital signal processor. The performance comparison of block algorithms is shown in Table 7.3.

Table 7.3. Performance comparison of non-overlapping block adaptive algorithms in terms of SNRI (dBs)

S. No.	Algorithm	Average SNRI for PLI Removal	Average SNRI for BW Removal	Average SNRI for MA Removal	Average SNRI for EM Removal
1.	BLMS	8.2149	3.4901	5.2423	3.8171
2.	FBLMS	19.2428	15.8662	15.9587	15.9646
3.	BNLMS	9.0584	3.9546	5.7237	4.2078
4.	**FBNLMS**	**20.3706**	**16.7628**	**16.6132**	**16.7681**
5.	BENLMS	10.5604	4.1781	6.1109	4.5390
6.	**FBENLMS**	**22.5811**	**17.7085**	**17.6163**	**17.7103**

Table 7.4. Performance comparison of overlapping block adaptive algorithms in terms of SNRI (dBs)

S. No.	Algorithm	Average SNRI for PLI Removal	Average SNRI for BW Removal	Average SNRI for MA Removal	Average SNRI for EM Removal
1.	**BBNSRLMS**	**10.2133**	**7.8046**	**8.4555**	**8.5012**
2.	BBNSLMS	8.1431	6.6569	6.6847	6.7352
3.	BBNSSLMS	8.8000	5.4971	5.7096	6.0536
4.	**BBENSRLMS**	**11.5130**	**9.4028**	**10.2293**	**10.3788**
5.	BBENSLMS	9.1737	7.2069	8.4736	7.6325
6.	BBENSSLMS	8.2808	6.3068	7.5022	6.7922

Next, we employed overlapping block processing using the BBNLMS and BBENLMS discussed in Chapter 4. To reduce computational complexity, we successfully developed ANCs using sign-based versions of both BBNLMS and BBENLMS. Of the two, BBNLMS had the better performance in terms of SNRI, EMSE and M_{ad}. Among the six sign-based algorithms BBENSRLMS performed best, followed by BBNSRLMS and then BBNSLMS, BBNSSLMS, BBENSLMS and BBENSSLMS in the order. From the simulation results it is clear that the proposed ANCs remove non-stationary noise efficiently. The proposed treatment provides high signal to noise ratio and lower computational complexity, making sign-based algorithms particularly suitable for wireless telecardiology systems. A comparison of overlapping block algorithms is shown in Table 7.4.

For work to reduce computational complexity and increase SNRI, we have chosen ANCs based on BBNSRLMS and BBENSRLMS for implementation in a real time environment on an embedded processor.

7.5. Review of Experimental Results on Embedded Processor

As described in Chapter 6, the eight chosen ANCs (and the conventional LMS based ANC) were implemented on a TI TMS320C6713. Of the 42 algorithms discussed in this work, SRLMS, SRDZLMS, NSRLMS, ENSRLMS, BBNSRLSM, BBENSRLMS, FLMS and FENLMS were chosen because they performed better than the others with respect to SNRI, computational complexity and would therefore be best suited for real time biotelemetry applications. For this all the eight algorithms written in MATLAB are rewritten in C language for processor implementation. Using the dataset of five signals, with 4000 samples we have performed the experiments for 10 times and average values are tabulated. For standardization of the results conventional LMS based noise canceller is developed and compared with the newly developed adaptive noise cancellers for ECG enhancement. The SNRI contrast of various algorithms is compared in Table 7.5.

From Table 7.5, it can be concluded that,

1. The experimental and simulation studies are well in match.
2. The newly developed ANCs are functioning effectively in reducing the artefacts PLI, BW, MA and EM along with channel noise.

Table 7.5. Performance comparison of various algorithms implemented on embedded DSP in terms of SNRI (dBs)

S. No	Algorithm	Average SNRI for PLI Removal		Average SNRI for BW Removal		Average SNRI for MA Removal		Average SNRI for EM Removal	
		Simulation	Experimental	Simulation	Experimental	Simulation	Experimental	Simulation	Experimental
1.	LMS	7.2741	6.8760	3.4080	3.2199	4.6154	4.3807	3.9484	3.6172
2.	SRLMS	6.9250	6.4814	2.5390	2.3068	3.5043	3.2364	2.8020	2.3165
3.	DZSRLMS	6.4173	6.0286	4.5439	4.3015	4.8520	4.4197	4.8700	4.2942
4.	NSRLMS	10.8815	10.4281	11.1317	10.7632	10.3672	9.9750	12.2121	11.5380
5.	ENSRLMS	9.5042	9.1257	9.9608	8.9841	9.5483	9.0421	10.2890	9.3927
6.	BBNSRLMS	10.0526	9.7843	9.3007	8.4590	8.6025	8.1637	10.2849	9.3574
7.	BBENSRLMS	10.6998	10.2584	10.1198	9.7987	10.1530	9.7591	11.5198	10.6911
8.	FBNLMS	18.8638	18.3027	13.5793	12.8672	15.9532	14.1786	13.3706	12.4572
9.	FBENLMS	21.0837	20.5203	14.7234	14.3511	16.0748	15.2355	14.5783	13.3190

7.6. Review of Conclusion

The above discussions lead to the following conclusions:

1. When PLI only is present, the LLMS based ANC performs better than other LMS weight update variants. SRLLMS achieves SNRI close to that of LLMS and SRLLMS needs only one multiplication to compute the weight update equation. Among all normalized algorithms, NSRLMS filters PLI efficiently. Of the block processing algorithms, frequency domain FBENLMS processing increases ECG signal resolution in terms of SNRI.
2. DZLMS effectively removes BW noise, and its SR version also achieves SNRI close to DZSRLMS, but with only one multiplication. Of the normalized algorithms, NSRLMS performs efficiently, and in block processing FBENLMS achieves highest SNRI.
3. The LMF algorithm cancels MA noise well, and DZLMS achieves an SNRI very close to it. Of the two, SRDZLMS achieves a better SNRI than SRLMF does. Among the normalized algorithms, NSRLMS achieves the highest SNRI, and among the frequency domain algorithms, FBENLMS is the best performer.
4. The LMF algorithm is also best at EM noise, and SRDZLMS is also a strong performer. Of the normalized algorithms NSRLMS achieves the highest SNRI, and FBENLMS is the best performing frequency domain algorithm.

From the literature, it is evident that all four artefacts are usually present in EDCG signals obtained under normal practical conditions. Our work suggests that the NSRLMS algorithm in time domain and the FBENLMS algorithm in the frequency domain, are capable to filter all artefact types, and are thus suitable for use in clinical practice.

7.7. Scope of Future Work

In this work, we have developed and proved the effectiveness of the adaptive filtering techniques for removing artefacts from cardiac signals in biotelemetry applications. It is however, felt that there may exist considerable scope for extending the work reported here along various directions for future investigations. These are briefly outlined below.

- This work has concentrated on the LMS based ANCs for ECG enhancement primarily by removing PLI, BW, MA and EM noises. Further ANCs development is needed to cancel other noise types like fetal noise, donor heart noise, pacemaker noise etc.
- For practical implementation of the developed ANCs, we used the TI TMS320C6713, but they can also be implemented with other digital signal processors or field programmable gate arrays (FPGAs).
- The practice of fewer leads to extract the signals for modern ECG recorders may lead to processing errors that can be removed by new algorithms, yet to be developed.
- There is scope for the development of intelligent cardiac systems. In which several algorithms can be used, depending upon the noise characteristics the suitable adaptive algorithm activates for filtering.
- New ANCs using neural networks and fuzzy logic can also be developed.

References

[1] I. S. N. Murthy, M. R. Rangaraj, K. Jaya Ram and A. K. Goyal, "Homomorphic Analysis and Modeling of ECG Signals," *IEEE Transactions on Biomedical Engineering*, vol. BME-26, no. 6, pp. 330-344, June, 1979.

[2] James C. Huhta and John G. Webster, "60-Hz Interference in Electrocardiography," *IEEE Transactions on Biomedical Engineering*, vol. BME-20, no. 2, pp. 91-101, March, 1973.

[3] J. A. Van Alste and T. S. Schilder, "Removal of base-line wander and power-line interference from the ECG by an efficient FIR filter with a reduced number of taps," *IEEE Transactions on Biomedical Engineering*, vol. 32, no. 12, pp. 1052-1060, 1985.

[4] Rik Vullings, Bert de Vries, and Jan W. M. Bergmans, "An Adaptive Kalman Filter for ECG Signal Enhancement," *IEEE Transactions on Biomedical Engineering,* vol. 58, no. 4, pp. 1094-1103, April, 2011.

[5] O. Sayadi and M. B. Shamsollahi, "Model-based fiducial points extraction for baseline wander electrocardiograms," *IEEE Transactions on Biomedical Engineering*, vol. 55, no. 1, pp. 347-351, Jan., 2008.

[6] Qinghua Zhang, A. I. Manriquez, C. Mdigue, Y. Papelier, and Michel Sorine, "An Algorithm for Robust and Efficient Location of T-Wave Ends in Electrocardiograms," *IEEE Transactions on Biomedical Engineering*, vol. 53, no. 12, pp. 2544-2552, Dec., 2006.

[7] F. Zhang and Yong. L, “QRS Detection Based on Multiscale Mathematical Morphology for Wearable ECG Devices in Body Area Networks,” *IEEE Transactions on Biomedical Circuits and Systems*, vol. 3, no. 4, pp. 220-228, August, 2009.

[8] Min Shao, Kenneth E. Barner and Michael H. Goodman, “An Interference Cancellation Algorithm for Noninvasive Extraction of Trans abdominal Fetal Electroencephalogram (TaFEEG),” *IEEE Transactions on Biomedical Engineering*, vol. 51, no. 3, pp. 471-483, March, 2004.

[9] K. C. Lai and John J. Shynk, “A Successive Cancellation Algorithm for Fetal Heart-Rate Estimation Using an Intrauterine ECG Signal,” *IEEE Transactions on Biomedical Engineering*, vol. 49, no. 9, pp. 943- 954, Sept., 2002.

[10] P. Sun, Q. H. Wu , A. M. Weindling, A. Finkelstein, and K. Ibrahim, “An Improved Morphological Approach to Background Normalization of ECG Signals,” *IEEE Transactions on Biomedical Engineering*, vol. 50, no. 1, pp. 117-121, Jan., 2003.

[11] Reza Sameni, Gari D. Clifford, Christian Jutten, and M. B. Shamsollahi, “Multichannel ECG and Noise Modeling: Application to Maternal and Fetal ECG Signals,” *Eurasip Journal on Advances in Signal Processing*, vol. 2007, Article ID 43407, 14 pages.

[12] N. V. Thakor and Yi-Sheng Zhu, “Applications of adaptive filtering to ECG analysis: noise cancellation and arrhythmia detection,” *IEEE Transactions on Biomedical Engineering*, vol. 38, no. 8, pp. 785-794, August, 1991.

[13] B. Widrow, J. Glover, J. M. McCool, J. Kaunitz, C. S. Williams, R. H. Hearn, J. R. Zeidler, E. Dong, and R. Goodlin, “Adaptive noise cancelling: Principles and applications,” *Proc. IEEE*, vol. 63, pp. 1692-1716, Dec. 1975.

[14] Mark Yelderma, Bernard Widro, John M Cioffi, Edward Hesler and Jeffrey A. Leddy, “ ECG Enhancement by Adaptive Cancellation of Electrosurgical Interference,” *IEEE Transactions on Biomedical Engineering*, vol. BME-30, no. 7, pp. 392-398, July, 1983.

[15] V. Almenar and A. Albiol, "A new adaptive scheme for ECG enhancement," *Signal Processing*, vol. 75, pp. 253-263, 1999.

[16] C. Vaz and N. V. Thakor, "Adaptive Fourier estimation of time-varying evoked potentials," *IEEE Transactions on Biomedical Engineering*, vol. 36, no. 4, pp. 448-455, April, 1989.

[17] A. K. Barros and N. Ohnishi, "MSE behavior of biomedical event-related filters," *IEEE Transactions on Biomedical Engineering*, vol. 44, no. 9, pp. 848-855, Sept. 1997.

[18] Floris Ernst, A. Schlaefer, S. Dieterich and A. Schweikard "A Fast Lane Approach to LMS prediction of respiratory motion signals," *Biomedical Signal Processing and Control*, vol. 3, pp. 291-299, 2008.

[19] C. Marque, C. Bisch, R. Dantas, S. Elayoubi, V. Brosse, C. Perot, "Adaptive filtering for ECG rejection from surface EMG recordings," *Journal of Electromyography and Kinesiology*, vol. 15, pp. 310-315, 2005.

[20] Patrick S. Hamilton, "A Comparison of Adaptive and Non adaptive Filters for Reduction of Power Line Interference in the ECG," *IEEE Transactions on Biomedical Engineering*, vol. 43, no. 1, pp. 105-109, Jan., 1996.

[21] S Tiinanen, M Tulppo, and T Seppänen, "Reducing the Effect of Respiration in Baroreflex Sensitivity Estimation With Adaptive Filtering," *IEEE Transactions on Biomedical Engineering,* vol. 55, no. 1, pp. 51-59, Jan., 2008.

[22] Ziarani. A. K and Konrad. A, "A nonlinear adaptive method of elimination of power line interference in ECG signals," *IEEE Transactions on Biomedical Engineering*, vol. 49, no. 6, pp. 540-547, June, 2002.

[23] Suzanna M. M. Martens, Massimo Mischi, S. Guid Oei, and Jan W. M. Bergmans, "An Improved Adaptive Power Line Interference Canceller for Electrocardiography," *IEEE Transactions on Biomedical Engineering*, vol. 53, no. 11, pp. 2220-2231, Nov., 1996.

[24] Omid Sayadi and M. B. Shamsollahi, "Multiadaptive BionicWavelet Transform: Application to ECG Denoising and Baseline Wandering

Reduction," *Eurasip Journal on Advances in Signal Processing*, vol. 2007, Article ID 41274, 11 pages.

[25] Y. Der Lin and Y. Hen Hu, "Power-line interference detection and suppression in ECG signal processing," *IEEE Transactions on Biomedical Engineering*, vol. 55, no. 1, pp. 354-357, Jan., 2008.

[26] U. Irusta, J. Ruiz, S. R. Gauna, T. Eftestøl, and J. Kramer-Johansen, "A Least Mean-Square Filter for the Estimation of the Cardiopulmonary Resuscitation Artifact Based on the Frequency of the Compressions, " *IEEE Transactions on Biomedical Engineering,* vol. 56, no. 4, pp. 1052-1062, April, 2009.

[27] S. Olmos and P. Laguna, "Steady-state MSE convergence analysis in LMS adaptive filters with deterministic reference inputs for biomedical signals," *IEEE Transaction on Signal Processing*, vol. 48, pp. 2229-2241, Aug. 2000.

[28] S. Olmos, L. Sornmo and P. Laguna, "Block adaptive filter with deterministic reference inputs for event-related signals: BLMS and BRLS," *IEEE Transaction on Signal Processing*, vol. 50, pp. 1102-1112, May, 2002.

[29] S. Poornachandra and N. Kumaravel, "Subband-Adaptive Shrinkage for Denoising of ECG Signals," *Eurasip Journal on Applied Signal Processing*, vol. 2006, Article ID 81236, Pages 1-9.

[30] Jacek M Leski and Norbert Henzel, "ECG baseline wander and power line interference reduction using nonlinear filter bank," *Signal Processing*, vol. 85, pp. 781-793, 2005.

[31] M. Ali Tinati and B. Mozaffary, "A Wavelet Packets Approach to Electrocardiograph Baseline Drift Cancellation," *Eurasip International Journal of Biomedical Imaging*, vol. 2006, Article ID 97157, Pages 1-9.

[32] Georgy. M and I. Dotsinsky, "Power-line interference elimination from ECG in case of non-multiplicity between the sampling rate and the power-line frequency," *Biomedical Signal Processing and Control*, vol. 3, pp. 334-340, 2008.

[33] A. K. Barros, M. Yoshizawa, and Y. Yasuda, “Filtering non correlated noise in impedance cardiography,” *IEEE Transactions on Biomedical Engineering*, vol. 42, pp. 324-327, Mar. 1995.

[34] Valentina D. A. Corino, Luca T. Mainardi, Martin Stridh, and Leif S ornmo, “Improved Time-Frequency Analysis of Atrial Fibrillation Signals Using Spectral Modeling,” *IEEE Transactions on Biomedical Engineering*, vol. 55, no. 12, pp. 2723-2730, Dec., 2008.

[35] T. Y. Ji, Z. Lu, Q. H. Wu and Z. Ji, “Baseline normalisation of ECG signals using empirical mode decomposition and mathematical morphology,” *Electronics Letters*, vol. 44 no. 2, 17th Jan., 2008.

[36] T. Pawar, S Chaudhuri, and S P. Duttagupta, “Body Movement Activity Recognition for Ambulatory Cardiac Monitoring,” *IEEE Transactions on Biomedical Engineering*, vol. 54, no. 5. pp. 874-882, May, 2007.

[37] S. R. Wiese, P. Anheier, R. D. Connemara, A. T. Mollner, T. F. Neils, J. A. Kahn, and J. G. Webster, “Electrocardiographic Motion Artifact Versus Electrode Impedance,” *IEEE Transactions on Biomedical Engineering*, vol. 52, no. 1, pp. 136-139, Jan., 2005.

[38] M. Izzetoglu, A. Devaraj, S. Bunce, and B. Onaral, “Motion Artifact Cancellation in NIR Spectroscopy Using Wiener Filtering,” *IEEE Transactions on Biomedical Engineering*, vol. 52, no. 5, pp. 934-938, May, 2005.

[39] P. Langley, E. J. Bowers, and A. Murray, “Principal Component Analysis as a Tool for Analyzing Beat-to-Beat Changes in ECG Features: Application to ECG-Derived Respiration,” *IEEE Transactions on Biomedical Engineering,* vol. 57, no. 4, pp. 821-829, April, 2010.

[40] F. C. Robertson, T. S. Douglas, and E. M. Meintjes, “Motion Artifact Removal for Functional Near Infrared Spectroscopy: A Comparison of Methods,” *IEEE Transactions on Biomedical Engineering*, vol. 57, no. 6, pp. 1377-1387, June, 2010.

[41] M. Lemay, J. M. Vesin, A. V. Osterom, V. Jacquemet, and L. Kappenberger, “Cancellation of Ventricular Activity in the ECG:

Evaluation of Novel and Existing Methods," *IEEE Transactions on Biomedical Engineering*, vol. 54, no. 3, pp. 542-546, March, 2007.

[42] K. Rheinberger, T. Steinberger, K. Unterkofler, M. Baubin, A. Klotz, and A Amann, "Removal of CPR Artifacts From the Ventricular Fibrillation ECG by Adaptive Regression on Lagged Reference Signals," *IEEE Transactions on Biomedical Engineering*, vol. 55, no. 1, pp. 130-137, Jan., 2008.

[43] T. Werther, Klotz, G. Kracher, M. Baubin, H. G. Feichtinger, H. Gilly, and A Amann, "CPR Artifact Removal in Ventricular Fibrillation ECG Signals Using Gabor Multipliers," *IEEE Transactions on Biomedical Engineering*, vol. 56, no. 2, pp. 320-327, Feb., 2009.

[44] A. Montazeri and J. Poshtan, "A Computationally Efficient Adaptive IIR solution to Active Noise and Vibration Control Systems," *IEEE Transactions on Automatic Control*, vol. 55, no. 11, pp. 2671-2676, November, 2010.

[45] Shou-Sheu Lin and Wen-Rong Wu, "A Low-Complexity Adaptive Echo Canceller for xDSL Applications," *IEEE Transactions on Signal Processing*, vol. 52, no. 5, pp. 1461-1465, May, 2004.

[46] J. Ramadhan M. "A New Adaptive Beam former for Optimal Acoustic Echo and Noise Cancellation with Less Computational Load," *IEEE, CCECE/CCGEI*, pp. 123-128, May 2008.

[47] M. Lee, B. Keum, Yunmok Son, Joo-Wan Kim, and Hwang Soo Lee, "A New Low-Complex Interference Cancellation Scheme for WCDMA Indoor Repeaters," *IEEE Region 8 SIBIRCON*, pp. 457-462, 2008.

[48] Georgi I. and K. Egiazarian, "Adaptive System for Noise Cancellation in Wireless Communications," *IEEE MELECON*, pp. 271-276, May 12-15, 2004.

[49] Hyun C. Shin, Ali H. Sayed and Woo-Jin Song, "Variable Step-Size NLMS and Affine Projection Algorithms," *IEEE Signal Processing letters*, vol. 11, no. 2, pp. 132- 135, Feb., 2004.

[50] L. R. Vega, Hernn Rey, Jacob Benesty and Sara Tressens, "A New Robust Variable Step-Size NLMS Algorithm," *IEEE Transaction on Signal Processing*, vol. 56, No. 5, pp. 1878-1893, May, 2008.

[51] C. Paleologu, Silviu Ciochina and Jacob Benesty, "Variable Step-Size NLMS Algorithm for Under-Modeling Acoustic Echo Cancellation," *IEEE Signal Processing letters*, vol. 15, pp. 5-8, 2008.

[52] Ching-An Lai "NLMS algorithm with decreasing step size for adaptive IIR filters," *Signal Processing*, vol. 82, pp. 1305-1316, 2002.

[53] Ahmed I. Sulyman and Azzedine Zerguine, "Convergence and steady-state analysis of a variable step-size NLMS algorithm," *Signal Processing*, vol. 83, pp. 1255-1273, 2003.

[54] Ning Li, Y. Zhang, Y. Hao and J. A. Chambers, "A new variable step-size NLMS algorithm designed for applications with exponential decay impulse responses," *Signal Processing*, vol. 88, pp. 2346-2349, 2008.

[55] Y. Zhang, Ning Li, Jonathon A. Chambers and A. H. Sayed, "Steady-State Performance Analysis of a Variable Tap-Length LMS Algorithm," *IEEE Transaction on Signal Processing*, vol. 56, no. 2, pp. 839-845, Feb., 2008.

[56] Y. N. Rao, D. Erdogmus, *Member,* and J. C. Principe, "Error Whitening Criterion for Adaptive Filtering: Theory and Algorithms," *IEEE Transactions on Signal Processing*, vol. 53, no. 3, pp. 1057-1069, March, 2005.

[57] J. Arenas-García, V. Gómez-Verdejo, and A. R. Figueiras-Vidal, "New Algorithms for Improved Adaptive Convex Combination of LMS Transversal Filters," *IEEE Transactions on Instrumentation and Measurement*, vol. 54, no. 6, pp. 2239-2249, Dec., 2005.

[58] K. Y. Hwang, and W. J. Song, "An Affine Projection Adaptive Filtering Algorithm with Selective Regressors," *IEEE Transactions on Circuits and Systems—II: Express Briefs*, vol. 54, no. 1, pp. 43-46, Jan., 2007.

[59] T. Moon, and T. Weissman, "Universal FIR MMSE Filtering," *IEEE Transactions on Signal Processing*, vol. 57, no. 3, pp. 1068-1083, March, 2009.

[60] M. S. E. Abadi and John H. Husoy, "Mean-square performance of the family of adaptive filters with selective partial updates," *Signal Processing*, vol. 88, pp. 2008-2018, 2008.

[61] J. Ni and F. Li, "A Variable Step-Size Matrix Normalized Subband Adaptive Filter," *IEEE Transactions on Audio, Speech and Language Processing*, vol. 18, no. 6, pp. 1290-1299, August, 2010.

[62] F. C. Souza, O. J. Tobias, R. Seara and D. R. Morgan, "A PNLMS Algorithm with Individual Activation Factors," *IEEE Transactions on Signal Processing,* vol. 58, no. 4, pp. 2036-2047, April, 2010.

[63] P. A. Regalia, "A Complex Adaptive Notch Filter," *IEEE Signal Processing Letters*, vol. 17, no. 11, pp. 937-940, Nov., 2010.

[64] Z. Ramadan, A. Poularikas "Performance Analysis of a New Variable Step-Size LMS Algorithm with Error Nonlinearities," *0-7803-8281-1/04, IEEE.* pp. 384-388, 2004.

[65] J. Boyle, N. Bidargaddi, A. Sarela, and M. Karunanithi, "Automatic Detection of Respiration Rate From Ambulatory Single-Lead ECG," *IEEE Transactions on Information Technology in Biomedicine*, vol. 13, no. 6, pp. 890-896, Nov., 2009.

[66] F. Sufi, Qiang. F., Ibrahim Khalil, and Seedahmed S. M, "Novel Methods of Faster Cardiovascular Diagnosis in Wireless Telecardiology," *IEEE Journal on Selected areas in Communications*, vol. 27, no. 4, pp. 537-552, May, 2009.

[67] F. Hu, Y. Xiao and Q. Hao, "Congestion-Aware, Loss-Resilient Bio-Monitoring Sensor Networking for Mobile Health Applications," *IEEE Journal on Selected Areas in Communications*, vol. 27, no. 4, pp. 450-465, May, 2009.

[68] Reza S. Dilmaghani, Hossein Bobarshad, M. Ghavami, Sabrieh Choobkar, and Charles Wolfe, "Wireless Sensor Networks for Monitoring Physiological Signals of Multiple Patients," *IEEE Transactions on Biomedical Circuits and Systems*, vol. 5, no. 4, pp. 347-356, August, 2011,

[69] C. H. Lin, S. T. Young, T. S. Kuo, "A remote data access architecture for home-monitoring health-care applications," *Medical Engineering & Physics*, vol. 29, pp. 199-204, March, 2006.

[70] F. Zhang and Y. Lian, "QRS Detection Based on Multiscale Mathematical Morphology for Wearable ECG Devices in Body Area Networks," *IEEE Transactions on Biomedical Circuits and Systems*, vol. 3, no. 4, pp. 220-228, August, 2009.

[71] A. Alesanco and J. Garcıa, "Clinical Assessment of Wireless ECG Transmission in Real-Time Cardiac Telemonitoring," *IEEE Transactions on Information Technology in Biomedicine*, vol. 14, no. 5, pp. 1144-1152, Sept., 2010.

[72] Jafar Ramadhan M., "Multi-Microphone Noise Reduction Technique Based on Up sampling and IIR-RLS Filter with less Computational Load," *IEEE International Conference on Intelligent and Advanced Systems*, pp. 1219-1223, 2007.

[73] K. Mayyas, and T. Aboulnasr, "Reduced-Complexity Transform-Domain Adaptive Algorithm with selective coefficient update," *IEEE Transactions on Circuits and Systems-II: Express Briefs*, vol. 51, no. 3, pp. 136-142, March, 2004.

[74] J. H. Zhang, J. F. Böhmeb, "Adaptive regularization network based neural modeling paradigm for nonlinear adaptive estimation of cerebral evoked potentials," *Medical Engineering & Physics* vol. 29, pp. 1008-1018, Oct., 2006.

[75] A. N. Ali, *Advanced Bio Signal Processing*. Berlin, Germany: Springer Verlag, 2009.

[76] K. Mayyas and Tyseer Aboulnasr, "Leaky LMS Algorithm: MSE Analysis for Gaussian Data," *IEEE Transactions on Signal Processing*, vol. 45, no. 4, pp. 927-934, April, 1997.

[77] O. J. Tobias, and R. Seara, "Leaky Delayed LMS Algorithm: Stochastic Analysis for Gaussian Data and Delay Modeling Error," *IEEE Transactions on Signal Processing*, vol. 52, no. 6, pp. 1596-1606, June, 2004.

[78] P. I. Hübscher, J. C. M. Bermudez, and V. H. Nascimento, "A Mean-Square Stability Analysis of the Least Mean Fourth Adaptive

Algorithm," *IEEE Transactions on Signal Processing*, vol. 55, no. 8, pp. 4018-4028, Aug., 2007.

[79] A. Zerguine, "Convergence and steady-state analysis of the normalized least mean fourth algorithm," *Digital Signal Processing*, vol. 17, no. 1, pp. 17-31, 2007.

[80] Williamson, G. A., Clarkson P. M, Sethares W A, "Performance Characteristics of the median adaptive filter," *IEEE Transactions on Acoustics, Speech and Signal Processing*, vol- ASSP-41. no. 2, pp. 667-680, Apr. 1993.

[81] Tyseer. A. and K. Mayyas, "A Robust Variable Step-Size LMS-Type Algorithm: Analysis and Simulations," *IEEE Transactions on Signal Processing.*, vol. 45, no. 3, pp. 631- 639, March, 1997.

[82] Wee-Peng Ang and B. Farhang-Boroujeny, "A New Class of Gradient Adaptive Step-Size LMS Algorithms," *IEEE Transactions on Signal Processing*, vol. 49, no. 4, pp. 805- 810, April, 2001.

[83] T. Aboulnasr and K. Mayyas, "A Robust Variable Step-Size LMS-Type Algorithm: Analysis and Simulations," *IEEE Transactions on Signal Processing*, vol. 45, No. 3, pp. 631- 639, March, 1997.

[84] Yonggang Zhang, Ning Li, Jonathon A. Chambers and Yanling Hao, "New Gradient-Based Variable Step Size LMS Algorithms," *Eurasip Journal on Advances in Signal Processing*, Article ID 529480, 9 pages, 2008.

[85] J. M. Grriz, J. Ramrez, S. C. Alvarez, C. G. Puntonet, E. W. Lang, and Deniz. E, "A Novel LMS Algorithm Applied to Adaptive Noise Cancellation," *IEEE Signal Processing Letters*, vol. 16, pp. 34-37, Jan, 2009.

[86] Farhang-Boroujeny, B., John Wiley and Sons, "*Adaptive Filters-Theory and Applications*," Chichester, UK, 1998.

[87] Eweda Eweda, "Comparison of RLS, LMS, and Sign Algorithms for Tracking Randomly Time-Varying Channels," *IEEE Transactions on Signal Processing*, vol. 42, no. 11, pp. 2937-2944, Nov., 1994.

[88] T. H. Park, D. H. Youn and I. W. Cha, "Multiplication-Free Adaptive Digital Filters," *Proceedings of IEEE* , vol. 76, no. 5, pp. 632-634, May, 1988.

[89] S. Dasgupta, J. S. Garnett, and C. R. Johnson, Jr., "Convergence of an Adaptive Filter with Signed Filtered Error," *IEEE Transactions on Signal Processing*, vol. 42, no. 4, pp. 946-950, April, 1994.

[90] R. Punchalard, J. Koseeyaporn and P. Wardkein, "Adaptive IIR notch filter using a modified sign algorithm," *Signal Processing*, vol. 89, pp. 239-243, 2009.

[91] Julie E. Greenberg, "Modified LMS Algorithms for Speech Processing with an Adaptive Noise Canceller," *IEEE Transactions on Speech and Audio Processing*, vol. 6, no. 4, pp. 338-351, July, 1998.

[92] Markus Rupp and Rudi Frenzel, "Analysis of LMS and NLMS Algorithms with delayed coefficient update under the presence of spherically invariant process," *IEEE Transactions on Signal Processing*, vol. 42, no. 3, pp. 668-672, March, 1992.

[93] Sethares, W. A, "Adaptive algorithms with nonlinear data and error functions," *IEEE Transactions on Signal Processing*, vol. 40, no. 9 , pp. 2199 – 2206, 1992.

[94] S. C. Douglas and Teresa H. Y. Meng, "Normalized Data Nonlinearities for LMS Adaptation," *IEEE Transactions on Signal Processing*, vol. 42, pp. 1352-1365, June, 1994.

[95] S. Jo, and S. W. Kim, "Consistent Normalized Least Mean Square Filtering With Noisy Data Matrix," *IEEE Transactions on Signal Processing*, vol. 53, no. 6, pp. 2112-2123, June, 2005.

[96] Ali H. Syed, John Wiley and Sons, "*Adaptive Filters*," New Jersey, USA, 2008.

[97] W. A. Sethares, Iven M. Y. Mareels, Briand. O. Anderson, C. Richard Johnson, and Robert R. Bitmead, "Excitation Conditions for Signed Regressor Least Mean Squares Adaptation," *IEEE Transactions on Circuits and Systems*, vol. 35, no. 6, pp. 613-624, June, 1988.

[98] Eweda Eweda, "Analysis and Design of a Signed Regressor LMS Algorithm for Stationary and Nonstationary Adaptive Filtering with Correlated Gaussian Data," *IEEE Transactions on Circuits and Systems*, vol. 37, no. 11, pp. 1367-1374, Nov., 1990.

[99] Shinichi Koike, "Analysis of Adaptive Filters Using Normalized Signed Regressor LMS Algorithm," *IEEE Transactions on Signal Processing*, vol. 47, no. 10, pp. 2710-2723, Oct., 1999.

[100] Haykin, S., *Adaptive Filter Theory*, Eaglewood Clirs, NJ: Prentice-Hall, 1986.

[101] Rangaraj M. Rangayyan, John Wiley and Sons, "*Biomedical Signal Analysis- A case study approach*," USA, 2002.

[102] Yin Zhou, Jialu Chen and Xiaodong Li, "A Time/Frequency-Domain Unified Delayless Partitioned Block Frequency-Domain Adaptive Filter," *IEEE Signal Processing letters*, vol. 14, no. 12, pp. 976-979, Dec., 2007.

[103] B. F. Boroujeny and K. S. Chan, "Analysis of the Frequency-Domain Block LMS Algorithm," *IEEE Transactions on Signal Processing*, vol. 48, no. 8, pp. 2332-2342, August, 2000.

[104] B. Rafaely, and S. J. Elliott, "A Computationally Efficient Frequency-Domain LMS Algorithm with Constraints on the Adaptive Filter," *IEEE Transactions on Signal Processing*, vol. 48, no. 6, pp. 1649-1655, June, 2000.

[105] D. H. Shin, R. H. Park, S. Yang, and J. H. Jung, "Block-Based Noise Estimation Using Adaptive Gaussian Filtering," *IEEE Transactions on Consumer Electronics*, vol. 51, no. 1, pp. 218-226, Feb., 2005.

[106] M. J. Narasimha, "Block Adaptive Filter With Time-Domain Update Using Three Transforms," *IEEE Signal Processing Letters*, vol. 14, no. 1, pp. 51-53, Jan., 2007.

[107] A. Mitra, "NLMS-based algorithm for decision feedback equalization," *Electronics Letters*, vol. 43 no. 25, 6th Dec., 2007.

[108] E. Walach and B. Widrow, "The least mean fourth adaptive algorithm and its family," *IEEE Transactions on Information Theory*, vol. 30, pp. 275–283, Feb 1984.

[109] Orlando Jos Tobias and Rui Seara, "Leaky-FXLMS Algorithm: Stochastic Analysis for Gaussian Data and Secondary Path Modeling Error," *IEEE Transactions on Speech and Audio Processing*, vol. 13, no. 6, pp. 1217-1230, Nov., 2005.

[110] *PhysioNet*, The Massachusetts Institute of Technology – Boston's Beth Israel Hospital (MIT-BIH) Arrhythmia Database, Available: http://www.physionet.org/physiobank/database/mitdb/ (Online).

[111] The MIT-BIH Normal Sinus Rhythm Database, *PhysioNet* .Available: http://www.physionet.org/physiobank/database/nstdb/ (Online).

[112] The MIT-BIH Noise Stress Test Database, *PhysioNet.* Available: http://www.physionet.org/physiobank/database/nstdb/ (Online).

[113] Paula S. R. Diniz, "*Adaptive Filtering, Algorithms and Practical Implementation,"* Third edition, Springer Publishers, 2008.

[114] N. J. Bershad, "Analysis of the Normalized LMS algorithm with Gaussian inputs," *IEEE Transactions on Speech and Audio Processing*, vol. ASSP-34, no. 4, pp. 793-805, Aug., 1986.

[115] S. C. Douglas,"A Family of Normalized LMS Algorithms," *IEEE Signal Processing Letters*, vol. 1, pp. 1352-1365, March,1994.

[116] N. J. Bershad, "Comments on 'comparison of the convergence of two algorithms for adaptive FIR digital filters," *IEEE Transactions on Acoustic, Speech, Signal Process.*, vol. ASSP-33, pp. 1604–1606, Dec. 1985.

[117] Parhi, K. K, "*VLSI Digital Signal Processing Systems,"* John Wiley and Sons, Inc., 1999.

[118] Rulph Chassaing, "*DSP Applications Using C and the TMS32OC6x DSK*," A Wiley-Inter science Publication John Wiley and Sons, Inc., 2002.

[119] Texas Instruments, *TMS320C6713 DSK Technical Reference*, 2004, http://c6000.spectrumdigital.com/dsk6713/V2/docs/dsk6713_TechRef.pdf.

[120] "*TMS320C6000 DSP/BIOS User's Guide*, SPRU303B," Texas Instruments, Dallas, TX, 2000.

[121] "*TMS320C6000 DSP/BIOS Application Programming Interface (API) Reference Guide SPRU403A*," Texas Instruments, Dallas, TX, 2000.

[122] Joseph D. Bronzing, *The Biomedical Engineering Handbook*, Published by CRC Press, 2000.

[123] Refet Firat Yazicioglu, Sunyoung Kim, Tom Torfs, Hyejung Kim, and Chris Van Hoof, "A 30 μW Analog Signal Processor ASIC for Portable Biopotential Signal Monitoring," *IEEE Journal of Solid-State Circuits*, vol. 46, no. 1, pp. 209-223, January, 2011.

[124] Tee Hui Teo, Xinbo Qian, Pradeep Kumar Gopalakrishnan, Yee Shan Hwan, Kuruveettil Haridas, Chin Yann Pang, Hyouk-Kyu Cha, Minkyu Je, "A 700-μW Wireless Sensor Node SoC for Continuous Real-Time Health Monitoring," *IEEE Journal of Solid-State Circuits*, vol. 45, no. 11, pp. 2292-2299, November, 2010.

[125] Kyungtae Kang, Kyung-Joon Park, Jae-Jin Song, Chang-Hwan Yoon, and Lui Sha, "A Medical-Grade Wireless Architecture for Remote Electrocardiography," *IEEE Transactions on Information Technology in Biomedicine*, vol. 15, no. 2, pp. 260-266, March, 2011.

[126] Ismet Sahin, Nuri Yilmazer, and Marwan A. Simaan, "A Method for Subsample Fetal Heart Rate Estimation under Noisy Conditions," *IEEE Transactions on Biomedical Engineering*, vol. 57, no. 4, pp. 875-883, April, 2010.

[127] World Health Organization, "The World Health Report 2008," *World Health Organization,* Geneva, 2008. Available: http://www.who. int/whr/2008/whr08_en.pdf.

[128] L. Hadzievski, B. Bojovic, V. Vukcevic, P. Belicev, S. Pavlovic, Z. Vasiljevic-Pokrajcic, and M. Ostojic, "A Novel Mobile Transtelephonic System With Synthesized 12-Lead ECG," *IEEE Transactions on Information Technology in Biomedicine*, vol. 8, no. 4, pp. 428-438, December, 2004.

[129] Dewar D. Finlay, Chris D. Nugent, Mark P. Donnelly and Robert L. Lux, "Eigenleads: ECG Leads for Maximizing Information Capture and Improving SNR," *IEEE Transactions on Information Technology in Biomedicine*, vol. 14, no. 1, pp. 428-438, January, 2010.

[130] SangJoon Lee, Jungkuk Kim and Myoungho Lee, "A Real-Time ECG Data Compression and Transmission Algorithm for an e-Health

Device," *IEEE Transactions On Biomedical Engineering*, vol. 58, no. 9, pp. 2448-2454, September 2011.

[131] Claudio De Capua, Antonella Meduri, and Rosario Morello, "A Smart ECG Measurement System Based on Web-Service-Oriented Architecture for Telemedicine Applications," *IEEE Transactions on Instrumentation and Measurement*, vol. 59, no. 10, pp. 2530-2538,October, 2010.

[132] P Raphisak, S. C. Schuckers and Jongh Curry, "An Algorithm for EMG Noise Detection in Large ECG Data," *Computers in Cardiology*, vol. 31, pp. 369-372, 2004.

[133] Yunfeng Wu, Rangaraj M. Rangayyan, Yachao Zhou and Sin-Chun Ng, "Filtering electrocardiographic signals using an unbiased and normalized adaptive noise reduction system," *Medical Engineering & Physics, Elsevier*, vol. 31, pp. 17-26, 2009.

[134] Manuel B. V., Binwei Weng and K. E. Barner, "ECG Signal denoising and baseline wander correction based on the empirical mode decomposition," *Computers in Biology and Medicine, Elsevier*, vol. 38, pp. 1-13, 2008.

[135] Chin-Teng Lin, Kuan-Cheng Chang, Chun-Ling Lin, Chia-Cheng Chiang, Shao-Wei Lu, Shih-Sheng Chang, Bor-Shyh Lin, Hsin-Yueh Liang, Ray-Jade Chen, Yuan-Teh Lee, and Li-Wei Ko, "An Intelligent Telecardiology System using a Wearable and Wireless ECG to Detect Atrial Fibrillation," *IEEE Transactions on Information Technology in Biomedicine*, vol. 14, no. 3, pp.726-733, May, 2010.

[136] B. Boucheham, Y. Ferdi and M. C. Batouche, "Piecewise linear correction of ECG baseline wander: a curve simplification approach," *Computer Methods and Programs in Biomedicine, Elsevier*, vol. 78, pp. 1-10, 2005.

[137] Piotr Augustyniak, "Autoadaptivity and Optimization in Distributed ECG Interpretation," *IEEE Transactions on Information Technology in Biomedicine*, vol. 14, no. 2, pp. 394-400, March, 2010.

[138] D. A. Tong, K. A. Bartels, and K. S. Honeyager, "Adaptive Reduction of Motion Artifact In The Electrocardiogram,"

Proceedings of the Second Joint EMBSBMES Conference, pp. 1403-1404, 2002.

[139] Shen Luo, Willis J. Tompkins, "Experimental Study: Brachial Motion Artifact Reduction in the ECG," *Computers in Cardiology*, pp. 33-36, 1995.

[140] M. Milanesi, N. Martini, N. Vanello, V. Positano, M. F. Santarelli, R. Paradiso, D. De Rossi, L. Landini, "Multichannel Techniques for Motion Artifacts Removal from Electrocardiographic Signals," *Proceedings of the 28th IEEE EMBS Annual International Conference*, pp. 3391-3394, September, 2006.

[141] Jianbo Gao, Hussain Sultan, Jing Hu, and Wen-Wen Tung, "Denoising Nonlinear Time Series by Adaptive Filtering and Wavelet Shrinkage: A Comparison," *IEEE Signal Processing Letters*, vol. 17, no. 3, pp. 237-240, March, 2010.

[142] V. D. A. Corino, L T. Mainardi, M Stridh, and L S Ornmo, "Improved Time–Frequency Analysis of Atrial Fibrillation Signals Using Spectral Modeling," *IEEE Transactions on Biomedical Engineering*, vol. 55, no. 12, pp. 2723-2730, Dec., 2008.

[143] World Health Organization Report, "Preventing Chronic diseases a vital investment," *World Health Organization*, Geneva, 2005. Available: http://www.who.int/chp/chronic_disease_report/en/.

[144] World Health Organization Report, "Prevention and control of non-communicable diseases: Implementation of global strategy," *World Health Organization*, Geneva, 2007. Available: https://apps.who.int/gb/ebwha/pdf_files/EB120/b120_22-en.pdf.

[145] World Health Organization Report, "Miscoding and misclassification of ischaemic heart disease mortality," *World Health Organization*, Geneva, 2001. Available: http://www.who.int/healthinfo/paper12.pdf

[146] World Health Organization Report, "Integrated management of cardiovascular risk," *World Health Organization*, Geneva, 2002. Available: http://whqlibdoc.who.int/publications/9241562242.pdf.

[147] Cromwell, L., Weibell, F. J., and Pfeiffer, E. A., "*Biomedical Instrumentation and Measurements*" Prentice-Hall, 1980.

[148] N. F. Guler and E. D. Ubeyli, "Theory and Applications of Biotelemetry," *Journal of Medical Systems*, vol. 26, no. 2, pp. 159-178, April, 2002.

[149] Jeutter, D. C., *Telecommunications for Health Care*, Biomedical Engineering Department, Marquette University. Available at http://www.eng.mu.edu/biotelem/objectives.html

[150] Kasten, C. K., *Telemetry is Coming of Age*. Available at http://www.raven1.net/telem1.htm.

[151] Mussivand, T., Hum, A., Holmes, K. S., and Keon, W. J., "Wireless monitoring and control for implantable rotary blood pumps," *Artif. Organs,* vol. 21, no.7, pp. 661–664, 1997.

[152] Meindl, J. D., and Ford, A. J., "Implantable telemetry in biomedical research," *IEEE Transaction on Biomedical Engineering*, vol. 31, no. 12, pp. 817–823, 1984.

[153] Guler, I., and Kara, S., "A low-cost biotelemetry system for long time monitoring of physiological data," *Journal of Medical Systems*, vol. 20, no. 3, pp. 151–156, 1996.

[154] D. Jabaudon, J. Sztajzel, K. Sievert, T. Landis, and R. Sztajzel, "Usefulness of Ambulatory 7-Day ECG Monitoring for the Detection of Atrial Fibrillation and Flutter After Acute Stroke and Transient Ischemic Attack," Stroke, *Journal of American Heart Association*, vol. 35, pp. 1647-1651, May, 2004.

[155] P. Chazal, S. Palreddy, and W.J. Tompkins, "Automatic Classification of Hearbeats Using ECG Morphology and Heartbeat Interval Features," *IEEE Transactions on Biomedical Engineering*, vol. 51, no. 7, pp. 1196-1206, Jul. 2004.

[156] Hyejung Kim, Refet Firat Yazicioglu, Tom Torfs, Patrick Merken, Chris Van Hoof and Hoi-Jun Yoo, "An Integrated Circuit for Wireless Ambulatory Arrhythmia Monitoring Systems," *31st Annual International Conference of the IEEE EMBS Minneapolis*, Minnesota, USA, pp. 5409-5412, September 2-6, 2009.

[157] R. Fensli, E. Gunnarson and T. Gundersen, "A Wearable ECG-recording System for Continuous Arrhythmia Monitoring in a

Wireless Tele-Home-Care Situation," *Proceedings of the 18th IEEE Symposium on Computer-Based Medical Systems*, June, 2005.

[158] N. Kalouptsidis and S. Theodoridis, *Adaptive System Identification and Signal Processing Algorithms*, Prentice Hall, New York, 1989.

[159] Michael Heiss, "Optimal Dead-Zone Characteristic for Minimizing the A-Posteriori Error in Basis Function Networks," *IEEE Proceedings of the 35th Conference on Decision and Control*, Kobe, Japan Dec., 1996, pp. 476-477.

[160] Michael Heiss, "Error-Minimizing Dead Zone for Basis Function Networks," *IEEE Transactions on Neural Networks*, vol. I, no. 6, Nov., 1996, pp. 1503-1506.

[161] Mark R. G. and Moody G. B., "The Impact of the MIT Arrhythmia Database," *IEEE Engineering in Medicine and Biology*, vol. 20, no. 3, June, 2001, pp. 45-50.

[162] Moody GB, Mark RG. The MIT-BIH Arrhythmia Database on CD-ROM and software for use with it. *Computers in Cardiology* 17:185-188, 1990.

[163] D. C. Reddy, *Biomedical Signal Processing Principles and Techniques*, Tata McGraw Hill, 2006.

[164] Elif Derya Übeyli, "Clinical Technologies: Concepts, Methodologies, Tools and Applications," Chapter 41, *Telemedicine and Biotelemetry for E-Health Systems*, pp. 676-692, IGI Publications, 2011.

[165] *Analog Devices products*, http://www.analog.com/en/processors-dsp/adsp-21xx/products/index.html#.

[166] *Texas Instruments DSP products*, http://www.ti.com/lsds/ti/dsp/home.page.

[167] *Freescale Semiconductors products*, http://www.freescale.com/webapp/sps/site/homepage.jsp?code=DSP-DSC_HOME.

[168] *Hyperstone processors*, http://www.hyperstone.com/.

[169] *VeriSilicon processors*, http://www.verisilicon.com/en/.

[170] *Analog Devices Mixed Signal DSP Controller, ADSP 21991 data sheets*, http://www.analog.com/static/imported-files/data_sheets/ADSP-21991.pdf.

[171] *Analog Devices Mixed Signal DSP Controller ADSP 21992 data sheets*, http://www.analog.com/static/imported-files/data_sheets/ADSP-21992.pdf.

[172] *Analog Devices ADSP 21362 data sheets*, http://www.analog.com/static/imported-files/data_sheets/ADSP-21362_21363_21364_21365_21366.pdf.

[173] *Analog Devices ADSP 21261 data sheets*, http://www.analog.com/static/imported-files/data_sheets/ADSP-21261_21262_21266.pdf.

[174] *Texas Instruments, TMS320C5515 Technical Reference*, http://www.ti.com/lit/ds/sprs645e/sprs645e.pdf

[175] *Texas Instruments, TMS320C5505 Technical Reference*, http://support.spectrumdigital.com/boards/evm5505/revd/files/EVM5505_TechRef_revd.pdf.

[176] *Texas Instruments, TMS320C6711 Technical Reference*, http://www.ti.com/lit/ds/sprs088o/sprs088o.pdf.

[177] *Freescale Semiconductor data sheet MSC8151*, http://cache.freescale.com/files/dsp/doc/data_sheet/MSC8151.pdf.

[178] *Freescale Semiconductor data sheet MSC8251*, http://cache.freescale.com/files/dsp/doc/data_sheet/MSC8251.pdf.

[179] *Hyperstone E1-32XSR data sheet*, http://www.hyperstone.com/en/Product-main-processor-features-E1-family-Hyperstone-USA-13,851.html.

[180] *VeriSilicon ZSP 400 data sheet*, http://www.verisilicon.com/vsi/vsiadmin/upfile/zsp400_pb.pdf.

[181] Jameson, J. N. St C.; Dennis L. Kasper; Harrison, Tinsley Randolph; Braunwald, Eugene; Fauci, Anthony S.; Hauser, Stephen L; Longo, Dan L, *"Harrison's principles of internal medicine,"* McGraw-Hill Medical Publishing Division, New York, ISBN: 0-07-140235-7, 2005.

[182] McMurray JJ and Pfeffer MA, "Heart failure," *Lancet* 365 (9474), DOI:10.1016/S0140-6736(05)66621- 4, pp. 1877–89, 2005.

[183] Steven Hollenberg and Stephen Heitner, *"Cardiology in Family Practice: A practice guide,"* Humana Press, 2011.

[184] Robert O'Rourke, Valentin Fuster and R W Alexander, *"Hurst's The Heart Manual of Cardiology,"* McGraw Hill Publications, 10th edition, 2001.

[185] Brian P. Griffin and Eric J. Topol, *"Manual of Cardiovascular Medicine,"* Lippincott Williams & Wilikins Publications, 2000.

[186] Elias Hanna and Roberto Quintal, *"Cardiology: Handbook for Clinicians,"* Scrub Hill Press, 2009.

[187] *Code Composers Studio User's Guide, SPRU328B*, Texas Instruments, Dallas, TX, 2000.

[188] *Code Composers Studio User's Guide, SPRU509*, Texas Instruments, Dallas, TX, 2001.

[189] *TMS320C6000 Code Composer Studio Tutorial, SPRU301C*, Texas Instruments, Dallas, TX, 2000.

AUTHOR CONTACT INFORMATION

Md. Zia Ur Rahman, PhD
Department of Electronics and Communication Engineering
Koneru Lakshmaiah Education Foundation
Green Fields, Vaddeswaram, Guntur, India
Email: mdzr55@gmail.com; mdzr@kluniversity.in

INDEX

A

B

C

D

E

F

H

I

L

M

T

V

W

The Essential Guide to Magnetic Resonance

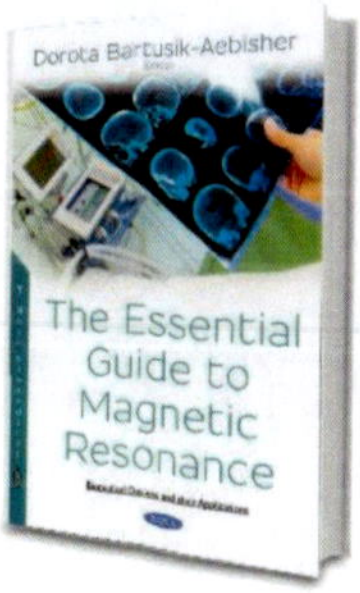

Editor: Dorota Bartusik-Aebisher

Series: Biomedical Devices and their Applications

Book Description: The opening chapter of The Essential Guide to Magnetic Resonance presents applications of Fluorine-19 Magnetic Resonance Imaging (19F MRI) in cancer research, tissue metabolomics, quantification of drug delivery, cellular tracking, tissue pH measurements and detection of 19F labeled cells.

Softcover ISBN: 978-1-53613-520-6
Retail Price: $82

Advances in Radiometry Research

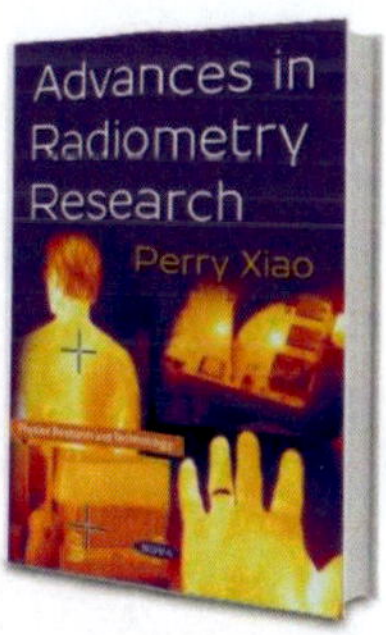

Author: Perry Xiao, Ph.D.

Series: Biomedical Devices and their Applications

Book Description: This book is intended to provide readers the theoretical background of radiometry, a resource of the latest radiometry technology, as well as the latest research in radiometry.

Hardcover ISBN: 978-1-53614-726-1
Retail Price: $230

Mechanical Ventilation: Applications, Technologies and Ethical Issues

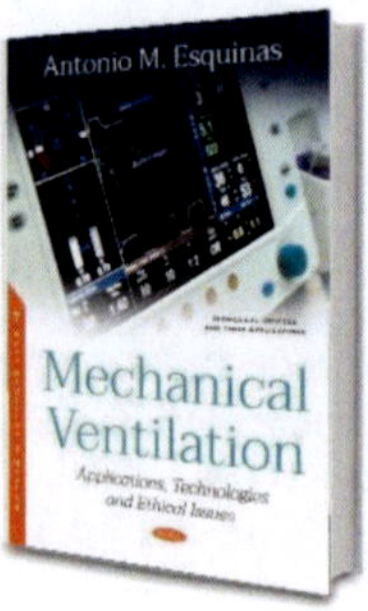

Editor: Antonio M. Esquinas

Series: Biomedical Devices and their Applications

Book Description: This book has made a selection of the hot topics about indications of mechanical ventilation, technological development advances, ethical and cost associated with mechanical ventilation.

Hardcover ISBN: 978-1-53615-002-5
Retail Price: $230